The Trainee's Companion to General Practice

For Churchill Livingstone:

Publisher: Lucy Gardner
Production Controller: Mark Sanderson
Sales Promotion Executive: Marion Pollock

The Trainee's Companion to General Practice

Edited by

Joe Rosenthal BSc MB BCh DRCOG MRCGP
Lecturer in General Practice, Department of Public Health and Primary Care, Royal Free Hospital School of Medicine, London, UK

Jeannette Naish MSc MBBS FRCGP
Senior Lecturer in General Practice, Department of General Practice and Primary Care, Joint Medical Colleges of St Bartholomew's and the London Hospitals, London, UK

Margaret Lloyd BSc MD FRCP MRCGP
Senior Lecturer in General Practice, Department of Public Health and Primary Care, Royal Free Hospital School of Medicine, London, UK

Foreword by
Alastair G. Donald OBE MA FRCPE FRCGP
President of the Royal College of General Practitioners

CHURCHILL LIVINGSTONE
EDINBURGH LONDON MADRID MELBOURNE NEW YORK AND TOKYO 1994

CHURCHILL LIVINGSTONE
Medical Division of Longman Group UK Limited

Distributed in the United States of America by Churchill Livingstone Inc., 650 Avenue of the Americas, New York, N. Y. 10011, and by associated companies, branches and representatives throughout the world.

© Longman Group UK Limited 1994

All rights reserved. No part of this publication may be reproduced, stored in a retrieval system, or transmitted in any form or by any means, electronic, mechanical, photocopying, recording or otherwise, without either the prior permission of the publishers (Churchill Livingstone, Robert Stevenson House, 1-3 Baxter's Place, Leith Walk, Edinburgh EH1 3AF), or a licence permitting restricted copying in the United Kingdom issued by the Copyright Licensing Agency Ltd, 90 Tottenham Court Road, London W1P 9HE.

First published 1994

ISBN 0-443-04703-0

British Library Cataloguing in Publication Data
A catalogue record for this book is available from the British Library.

Library of Congress Cataloging in Publication Data
A catalog record for this book is available from the Library of Congress.

The publisher's policy is to use **paper manufactured from sustainable forests**

Produced by Longman Singapore Publishers (Pte) Ltd
Printed in Singapore

Contents

Contributors vii
Foreword ix
Preface xi

SECTION 1
Introduction

1. The trainee year 3
   C. Donovan
2. Health not illness 25
   J. Horder

SECTION 2
In practice

3. Behind the scenes — how general practice is organised 49
   S. Brant
4. Communication in practice 105
   R. A. Savage
5. Disease prevention and health promotion in practice 137
   M. Lloyd
6. Clinical care in practice 189
   Part 1   Episodic care   —   *J. Naish, J. Rosenthal* 190
   Part 2   Continuing care   —   *J. Naish* 209
7. Audit and research in practice 237
   M. Lloyd

SECTION 3
The MRCGP and other examinations

8. The MRCGP examination 267
   J. Rosenthal
9. Diplomas for trainees 283
   J. Rosenthal
10. Further reading 291
    J. Rosenthal

Index 295

Contributors

Stephen Brant MSc MRCP MRCGP
General Practitioner, East Molesey, Surrey, UK

Chris Donovan MA MBBS DObstRCOG
General Practitioner, North London; Course Organiser, Royal Free Hospital and Bloomsbury Vocational Training Schemes, London, UK

John Horder CBE MD(Hon) FRCGP FRCP FRCPsych
Retired General Practitioner; Past President, Royal College of General Practitioners, London, UK

Margaret Lloyd BSc MD FRCP MRCGP
Senior Lecturer in General Practice, Department of Public Health and Primary Care, Royal Free Hospital School of Medicine, London, UK

Jeannette Naish MSc MBBS FRCGP
Senior Lecturer in General Practice, Department of General Practice and Primary Care, Joint Medical Colleges of St Bartholomew's and the London Hospitals, London, UK

Joe Rosenthal BSc MBBCh DRCOG MRCGP
Lecturer in General Practice, Department of Public Health and Primary Care, Royal Free Hospital School of Medicine, London, UK

Richard A. Savage MSc MRCGP DObstRCOG
General Practitioner, South London; Course Organiser, St Thomas' Hospital Vocational Training Scheme, London, UK

Foreword

Doctors who embark on a career in general practice are required to undertake a 3-year period of training after Registration, but only one of these years will normally be spent in general practice itself. The previous clinical educational experience will have been dominated by hospital-based specialties, modified only by instruction offered in a Department of General Practice or Community Medicine. The shift into the environment of general practice represents a major cultural change and there is a great deal to learn in a very short period of time if the doctor is to be adequately prepared to assume the full responsibilities of an independent general practitioner at the completion of his training.

Fortunately, appointments as trainee general practitioners are not part of a fixed establishment and therefore adequate time is available for educational activities of both a formal and informal nature allowing the trainee to expand a knowledge base relevant to general practice and to reflect on and try to understand the encounters with patients which are the basis of general practice.

Modern general practice involves a colossal range of activities of both a clinical and administrative nature. The clinical component ranges from an understanding of health and its promotion to the management of the full range of disease processes encountered in practice and the application to them of sophisticated modern remedies. The success of a modern practice also increasingly demands a knowledge of management and an understanding and use of a range of information technologies. Central, however, to all of these activities will be the ability to communicate successfully with patients, peers, and employed staff.

The Trainee's Companion to General Practice introduces the trainee to all of these areas of modern general practice, and will assist the trainee to make best use of the concentrated experience of the trainee practitioner appointment. It will act as a guide to the educational processes which have been perhaps more fully developed in general practice than in any other branch of medicine and will help the trainee to understand the complexities of the educational structure that supports these educational activities.

I am happy to commend this book to any doctor preparing for a career in general practice and I would encourage him or her to make full use of the resources available through the Royal College of General Practitioners, into whose membership the trainee will be welcomed at the successful completion of a period in practice which this book will help to make a fulfilling experience.

1993 A. G. Donald

Preface

This book has two closely related aims. Firstly, and as its name suggests, to provide a 'companion' for doctors who are new to general practice. The transition from hospital medicine to the wider world of primary health care can be a difficult one, and we hope to put up some signposts to help along the way. Secondly, to identify and explore the basic principles of general practice. A number of books supply guidance on 'how to do' general practice but few get to grips with the fundamental concepts upon which our work is based. We have tried to fill this gap.

As a result of these aims, what you will find within the pages that follow is a mixture of practical and theoretical, of concrete and abstract. Practical sections such as Chapter 3, which looks at the organisation of general practice, will help to make sense of the day-to-day work of the GP, while more reflective sections such as Chapter 2, examining the concept of 'health', are intended to promote thinking about the nature of our discipline.

The division of subject matter in Section 2 we hope will be useful but recognise to be artificial. It is inevitable that there will be some overlap between the issues presented in the different chapters.

We would like to thank our four contributors for their hard work, not just in supplying their individual chapters but also in sharing the thinking and planning behind the book. We are also grateful to trainees and colleagues who have read and criticised the material, to Lucy Gardner and the staff of Churchill Livingstone for their help and encouragement and to Elaine Harris for her efficient and good-humoured secretarial support. A special thank you goes to Janice Rymer of Guy's Hospital who really made it all happen in the first place.

We expect that this book will appeal primarily to GP trainees and their trainers but also hope that it may be of value to any GP taking a critical look at their work. It is far from our intention that this should be a 'textbook of general practice' which will contain the information to do the job. Rather we see it as providing a framework upon which to build during the trainee year and beyond.

J. Rosenthal
J. Naish
M. Lloyd

London 1993

SECTION 1

Introduction

1. The trainee year

Chris Donovan

INTRODUCTION

Joining a practice as a trainee is exciting, if somewhat daunting. It is only after years of preparation in hospital medicine that the doctor first practises in the setting they have chosen for their professional life. Entering general practice is very different from changing firms in hospital; almost everything is different — attitudes, daily routines, clinical problems, forms and patients' expectations, and even the hours of work. Doctors will know little about practising in the different environment of general practice and for this reason the idea of a trainee year alongside a recognised trainer was devised. The first point a trainee should accept is that, however competent they have been as a hospital doctor, there is much for them to learn in the new setting of general practice and the trainee year provides a wonderful opportunity for learning.

To be able to learn it is first necessary to recognise, and then to share, your areas of ignorance. This is not a comfortable process for anyone. Even the experienced GP cannot know everything and most patients are grateful when the doctor tells them that she or he needs to seek advice on a certain problem. Patients, receptionists, health visitors, nurses and GPs will generally be understanding when a trainee says she or he does need to learn more about a situation. Most people will be happy to help and answer questions. One trainer has written: 'Every trainee feels anxious when starting work in a new setting, which is quite different from hospital. We try to reduce the stresses as much as we can by creating an atmosphere in which the trainee plays a full part in everything that goes on.'

Most training practices are as understanding and the trainee will become quickly involved in many aspects of the practice.

CHOOSING A PRACTICE

Some trainees select a training practice without much thought. They approach the nearest practice to where they live and, being busy and tired in their hospital jobs, have little time to consider the pros and cons of joining a particular practice. Many are flattered and relieved when the first trainer they meet offers to take them on. Sometimes these doctors identify problems only once they have jointed a practice — they may not get on with their trainer, they may be overworked, they may have poor teaching and inadequate support.

At her interview Dr O found the partners in her local training practice very friendly. A month after joining she discovered that all visits were delegated to her and the other trainee. Moreover, no time was set aside for tutorials and instead she was expected to air her problems with her trainer if there was time over coffee at the end of surgery. Despite both trainees complaining, the situation did not improve. Dr O, not wishing to leave the practice or to upset her working relationships, accepted the position and completed her year, but she remained extremely unhappy.

The most important factor in the whole educational process of this year is the trainer/trainee relationship. Trainers undergo a rigorous process of selection and re-selection, but there will naturally be some who are more conscientious or better teachers than others.

To reduce the chance of encountering problems, the trainee needs to select a practice with care. It is not a bad idea to start the process a year or so before the appointment, given that many practices appoint their trainees well in advance. A list of trainers is available from the GP Regional Advisor's office and it may also be helpful to contact the local course organisers, the Regional Associate Advisors, past trainees or those in the middle of their year.

When choosing it must be remembered that the trainee will need to live relatively close to the practice when on-call during nights and weekends. Thus practices near to where the trainee lives should be considered first. Some trainees will, however, be prepared to commute in order to spend the year with a particular trainer in whom they have confidence, and they will need to find local accommodation to use when on call. Another factor influencing the choice of practice will be the area in which the trainee eventually wishes to practice. It is often easier to find an eventual partnership in an area where you are known as a result of your training year.

Once potential practices have been identified, the trainee will need to contact the trainer and arrange a visit to the practice. First impressions will tell the trainee whether they wish to proceed further. If they do, they should try and find out if there are any snags associated with a particular training practice. This can be done by talking to at least one preceding trainee, to the partners and to the practice administrator. The local course organiser may also be helpful. If all seems acceptable and the trainer is keen to make an appointment, it is then advisable to arrange to have a long talk with the trainer about the training year.

During this discussion several important considerations need to be covered.

Workload

All trainees are expected to be supernumerary to the running of the training practice. On the other hand, the trainee must receive wide clinical experience and be given the opportunity to carry responsibility throughout the year. It is important to ask the trainer about workload, the on-call rota, holidays and study leave, as well as opportunities for attending the half-day release course.

Tutorials

The trainee needs to ask how tutorials are organised and how much protected time is given to formal teaching. It is recommended that at least half a session each week should be set aside by trainer and trainee for tutorials. The attitude of other members of the practice to training, as well as the cover for the trainee within the practice, is also important.

Trainer's views of training and practice

It is essential for the trainee to establish if they are likely to get on with a prospective trainer. To do this, it is helpful to sit in and watch the trainer run a surgery, and to discuss the trainer's philosophy of training and practice, as well as the teaching methods they use.

Trainee's objectives for the year

The trainee should express their learning objectives for the year and identify areas in which they may feel lacking in confidence. They should also decide whether they intend to sit any further examinations such as the DCH, DRCOG or MRCGP. They may be keen to visit a rural or an inner city practice, or to undertake a certain project. Some trainees will wish to attend a study course to learn more about new areas such as counselling or family therapy.

If the prospective trainer is sympathetic to a doctor's objectives and they fit in with their own ideas for the year, a plan for the coming months should be drawn up bringing together all the objectives. At the same time plans for learning and assessment should be discussed and agreed, including perhaps starting a learning diary and completing rating scales (see later).

THE TRAINEE'S CONTRACT

Every trainee must have a signed contract with their employer, i.e. their trainer. At the time of applying to a practice, it may seem awkward to discuss the contract but this is necessary in case problems develop later in the year. It is also a learning experience since, when you become a principal, a contract or partnership agreement with the partners will need to be negotiated.

The BMA produces a sample contract and this can be the starting point for discussing important areas:

1. How much notice needs to be given if either party wishes to terminate the agreement
2. A description of the duties and responsibilities both of trainer and trainee
3. Holiday and study leave entitlement
4. The procedure for dealing with any dispute or if either party falls seriously ill
5. Arrangements for pay and superannuation (see below).

Dr M joined a practice without discussing or signing a contract. Early on the trainer discovered that she intended to continue her one session a week at the local hospital, with whom she had already signed a contract. Her trainer advised her that she was required to work full-time in the practice and that she should give up her hospital session. As she had not signed a contract with the trainer, she left the practice and continued her hospital session.

Financial considerations

The method of paying trainees is complicated. At first the trainee does not need to know all the details but they should establish the basic salary and when the first payment will be made. Most trainees will have been used to being paid monthly and therefore it is best to negotiate payment at the end of each month rather than quarterly, as most partners are paid.

Details of trainee and GP payment are given in the Statement of Fees and Allowances or 'Red Book' which should be sent to every trainee by their FHSA. The book is difficult to read but is worth studying as it describes the financial basis on which all general practices are founded. The following points should be noted:

1. The trainee's salary is related to the last NHS post held (salaries for work outside the NHS or abroad, and overtime pay for hospital work are not considered). On becoming a trainee the salary should rise to the next point on the incremental scale.

2. Removal expenses may be paid and the FHSA should be contacted if there is any disagreement about this.

3. It is not permitted for the trainer to make any additional payments to the trainee, and all fees earned by the trainee belong to the practice.

4. The trainee who wishes to undertake part-time work outside practice hours must first get permission from both the trainer and the FHSA.

5. A car allowance is not immediately deductible and must be declared to the tax inspector.

6. The cost of installing a new telephone or a bedside extension is reimbursable buy the FHSA.

In the event of sickness, the trainee will be paid for up to three months. It is wise therefore for a trainee to insure against sickness of longer than 3–4 months. If the trainee is away from the practice for more than 2 weeks due to sickness, the training year will need to be extended accordingly.

At the time of writing a woman trainee is only entitled to maternity leave if she has completed 12 months employment in the NHS immediately before applying for a trainee post. This rule is, however, due to change by early 1994 in line with EEC Regulations.

Expenses incurred when attending for interview with a trainer can be claimed from the FHSA, providing a job offer is not refused without 'good reason'.

SUMMARY BOX

Questions to consider when choosing a practice

- Will you 'get on' well with this trainer and this practice?
- Can you cover your 'on-call' duties?
- Have you sought local advice on the practice from past trainees, associate advisor and course organiser?
- Are you clear about:
  — workload
  — tutorial arrangements
  — the trainer's views on training?
- Have you discussed your objectives and ideas about assessment for the year and matched them with the trainer?
- Have you discussed and signed a contract?
- Do you know how much and when you will be paid?

PHASES OF THE TRAINEE YEAR

Preparation for the trainee year starts with the selection of a training practice and often continues during the first few days of the year. Pereira Gray has suggested that the training year can be divided into a total of five phases: preparation, adjustment, working phase, partnership phase, and the final phase (see Table 1.1).

During the year the trainee should develop independence and a tendency to practise hospital medicine should give way to a sense of identity as a GP.

Some trainees enter a 3-year vocational training scheme in which up to 3 months is spent with a trainer at the start and 9 months at the end, and the phases considered below in 1 year will be spread out.

Table 1.1 Phases of the training year

Phase	Time scale	Change in trainee
Preparation	Before starting and first week	Trainee dependence
Adjustment	First month	Trainee has a hospital outlook
Working phase	2–7 months	
Partnership	8–10 months	Trainee has developed a GP outlook
Final phase	10–12 months	Trainee autonomy

Adjustment

It takes around a month for the average trainee to adjust to working in general practice. The process of adjustment includes the preparation described above, the signing of the contract and shadowing the trainer. The latter involves sitting in on the trainer's surgeries, observing them in consultations and dealing with the practice paperwork and administration, and accompanying them on home visits. The trainee should also shadow and get to know other partners with whom they will be working because the whole practice forms the teaching environment for the year.

Other members of the team

Much can be learnt from sitting in the waiting area (before the trainee is recognised by the patients), where comments can be overheard about the surgery as seen from the patient's point of view. It can also be helpful to sit alongside the receptionist and from this an appreciation can be gained of their difficult task liaising between the doctors and their patients. The trainee can also observe how appointments are made and how visits are recorded, as well as getting to know the receptionists.

Many trainees find it helpful to accompany the district nurse and health visitor. This not only enables them to get to know these members of the GP team, but is also a lesson in the geography of the practice area and the role of their colleagues.

FHSA and other visits

The trainee may find it helpful early on to visit their local FHSA. The FHSA is responsible for administrating the district's general practices, opticians, dentists and pharmacists. From a visit the trainee will learn more about the many NHS forms and see them processed after they have left the practice.

Other helpful visits include the local pharmacist, social services and hospice.

After a busy and responsible job in hospital, this passive role, sitting watching others at work, can appear tedious, but most trainees look back on this as a useful learning period; it is the time when the foundation is laid for the work throughout the trainee year. It is also the time when word spreads among the patients that a new doctor has joined the practice, and this in itself may prompt them to consult the trainee and fill their surgeries when they begin. The trainee should start to see a few patients in their first weeks to appreciate the relevance of this phase and to banish boredom!

Points to learn in the first month

During this passive phase there are many functions specific to GP practice for the trainee to learn, including:

- how paperwork is dealt with, e.g. repeat prescriptions, temporary residents, and contraceptive, maternity and insurance forms
- how aspects of the 1990 Contract are dealt with, e.g. immunisation, paediatric surveillance, minor surgery, visits to the over 75s, cervical smears, etc. (see Ch. 3)
- to whom the partners refer their patients, both within the NHS and privately
- how to use the social and community services
- how the doctors work and communicate with the nurses, health visitors, social workers and others in the primary care team.
- how to use the practice computer system

This is also a time when the trainee can start to build a list of useful telephone numbers and become familiar with local geography. Some practices provide photographs of blocks of flats or enlarged maps to help the identification of unfamiliar roads. This prepares the trainee for when they are on-call. Shadowing partners on-call also prepares the trainee by showing them how to respond to emergencies, as well as how to contact their trainer should the need arise.

During the first month the trainer and trainee should start to plan the year in detail, perhaps during the weekly tutorials. A schedule will need to be planned if study leave is required, if the trainee is to undertake a specific project or if there are other objectives to be achieved during the year.

Starting a surgery

After a week or two of sitting in, the trainer will suggest that the trainee starts their own surgery. The receptionist will be asked to book in patients at relatively long intervals, which will give the trainee plenty of time to undertake their first consultations. At first the trainee will be heavily dependent on advice: what form to use?, how to manage a condition?, to whom should a patient be referred? This is also the time when the trainee should manage a few home visits on their own.

Many trainees find their new role awkward. They must adapt to working without a 'white coat' and all that entails. Patients may be disappointed that they cannot see their own GP or the previous trainee, and even, occasionally, may ask if you are qualified. The term 'trainee' has been criticised for this last reason but, as yet, no alternative has been widely adopted. Most trainees are relieved to be seeing patients on their own again and using their own clinical skills. They start to feel like a GP.

SUMMARY BOX

The first month

- Shadow trainer and partners
- Sit with receptionist
- Go out on visits with members of the primary care team
- Visit social services, local pharmacist, the FHSA, etc.
- Become familiar with practice forms and paperwork
- Note to whom partners refer their patients
- Build up a list of useful telephone numbers
- Get to know the local geography
- Prepare for 'on-call'— equipment, telephone, back-up, etc.
- Begin tutorials, day release and planning the year
- Begin your own surgery.

The working phase

Routine surgeries

Trainees may at first be apprehensive that patients may not choose to see them and are flattered when they do so. It is wise to be a little cautious. Some patients make a habit of booking to see the new trainee in the hope that they will get more doctor time, increased visits, easy referrals or more drugs. Also, the trainee may form too close a relationship with some patients early on and then may not be able to maintain these as the workload increases. The balance between patient dependency and responsibility with appropriate GP advice should be explored early on.

The appointment of a new doctor at any practice is an opportunity for a review of medical care. It is well known that new 'clinical eyes' identify new diagnoses and solutions that have previously been missed. The wise trainee will not gloat if they discover that Mrs Smith has hypothyroidism or Mr Brown has late onset diabetes which has gone unnoticed by the partners. Experienced GPs have their limitations and so will the trainee when they become established principals. Indeed, arriving straight from hospital, the trainee will be more familiar with many aspects of medical care. It should be remembered that the established GP will have vast experience to share with the trainee, and tact should be shown when the trainee does demonstrate advanced knowledge or skills to others in the practice.

Women trainees

Women trainees may at first be flattered when a lot of gynaecological problems and antenatal care come their way. However, there is a danger that these will soon swamp their practice and prevent them from seeing a mix of clinical problems. Most trainees will have completed six months in hospital obstetrics and gynaecology and already be proficient at dealing with these cases. They should continue to do so, but they also need learning opportunities in other areas, e.g. terminal care, asthma or dermatology. Women trainees should discuss their case mix with their trainer and explore ways of avoiding too many similar referrals. Reception staff may need to be briefed about maintaining a spread in appointments. Whatever the policy, the woman trainee needs to feel in control of the situation.

On-call

At the end of the adjustment phase, the trainee will join the on-call rota. Covering for the whole practice for a night or weekend can be a worrying prospect and in advance the trainee should discuss with their trainer how to handle emergencies: e.g. what is the practice policy for coronaries, acute asthma attacks, psychiatric emergencies, sudden death, etc? In fact, major problems are rare and most trainees cope well with their on-call duties. However, there should always be back-up available from a partner, and the trainee should use this facility if necessary.

Dr K was on-call during his second weekend at the practice. His trainer had a family wedding to attend, but had asked another local doctor to cover the trainee. The trainee was called by a patient who said she had found her husband dead on the kitchen floor. The trainee did not know how to handle the situation as he had not been taught to contact the Coroner's Officer. For a short time he debated what to do, and then, reluctantly, called the proxy trainer for help, and the situation was easily resolved.

Communication skills

All too quickly, the trainee will find that their week is filled with clinical work. Patients are booked in at shorter intervals, the number of visits increases, paperwork escalates. Patients will begin to view the trainee as their own doctor and turn to them for advice. In order to manage the mounting workload, the trainee may need to adapt and monitor their communication/consultation skills and also record-keeping skills. These should be discussed with the trainer or at the half-day release course, and useful advice can be found in the literature. Basic skills can be explored by videotaping consultations, role-play, or by the trainer observing the trainee in surgery.

Different clinical situations

During this phase the trainee should experience as many different clinical situations as possible. A crude categorisation of clinical situations is:

1. Emergency work, e.g. coronaries, psychiatric breakdown
2. 'Bread and butter' situations, e.g. URTI, vaginal discharge, skin complaints
3. Chronic conditions, e.g. multiple sclerosis, Parkinson's disease
4. Prevention/health promotion, e.g. well person and baby clinics.

For the trainee there is a danger of too much work falling within categories 1 and 2 at the expense of 3 and 4. The trainer should be asked to advise about gaining experience in the supervision of chronic conditions and health promotion clinics. Patients with ongoing conditions such as multiple sclerosis, diabetes, or dementia are often willing to be referred to the trainee. Many trainees welcome the opportunity of being introduced to a pregnant woman early on, so that during the year they will be able to follow her through to the birth. If there are any clinical areas in which the trainee particularly lacks confidence, these should be explored with the trainer so that some cases can be directed towards the trainee and their management discussed. One method of facilitating this is to share surgeries and to suggest that selected patients see the trainee at the next surgery; another is for the trainee to ask to be called in when other doctors see suitable patients.

It is tempting for the inexperienced trainee to fill the day with surgeries, clinics, visits and overlook the need to set aside time to reflect on and discuss clinical experience. Discussion can take place informally at the end of surgeries, within timetabled tutorials or case discussions, or at the half-day release course. It may be helpful for the trainee to continue to sit in during their trainer's surgery or vice versa. Some trainees prefer to video their consultations and discuss the recording with their trainer or with their peers and the course organiser at the half-day release course. The trainee should also consult the books and journals in the practice library.

The partnership phase

With experience the trainee will develop confidence in the role of GP. They may feel that they have changed their approach from that of

THE TRAINEE YEAR   13

> **SUMMARY BOX**
>
> **The working phase**
>
> Learning by doing and assessing progress is the essence of this phase.
> - Build up a list of patients seen in surgery, on visits and on call.
> - Gain experience in the full range of clinical situations
> - Review communication and recording skills and try to improve them
> - Discuss with others and read about clinical problems encountered
> - Discuss difficult clinical experiences at the half-day release
> - Discuss areas of ignorance in tutorials
> - Cooperate with the trainer in assessing knowledge, skills and attitude.

practising hospital medicine in a community setting to a different general practice style. Others feel lost while they are making this transition, which coincides with the time when the novelty of being a GP may have worn off and surgeries begin to appear repetitive and the paperwork tedious. Patients who do not improve may make the trainee feel increasingly frustrated. In short, the honeymoon period is over and the trainee's morale may slump. This disillusionment is so commonplace that it is almost to be expected, although it varies in degree with different personalities. Those areas which are troubling the trainee need to be explored and ways of coping with them identified if the next phase in the training is to begin.

No job is without its difficulties. Some trainees find certain patients particularly difficult to deal with, e.g. a forceful and demanding patient, a demented person or an attractive teenager. Other trainees are very upset by drug addicts, suicides or the terminally ill. The trainee should address particular problems by talking through them during tutorials or at the half-day release.

Dr F, a 27-year-old woman trainee, was consulted in her first week by a 28-year-old man. He was a muscular, fit-looking man who confided to her that he had never told any other GP that he was HIV positive. Despite being referred to the local AIDS clinic, he consulted the trainee regularly over the next few months. He developed full-blown AIDS and became emaciated and ill. Eventually he told the trainee he could not face a slow deterioration in health and had decided to hang himself. In describing the situation to the half-day release group, the trainee burst into tears and admitted that she admired and liked this patient, and did not know what to do. The group sympathised with the situation and supported the trainee, who was then able to continue seeing the patient and introduce him to further help.

The changing trainer-trainee relationship

As the trainee's confidence and competence grows, the relationship with the trainer will change. For most of the year the trainer is usually the dominant figure in the relationship. During the 'partnership phase' the relationship moves closer to that of colleagues or partners, and although assessment continues, the trainee is usually the more active in identifying areas of need and their solutions. The trainee may suggest that teaching arrangements are changed or that they visit another practice or attend a course. They may begin to discuss problems outside the practice, e.g. with the associate advisor or course organiser. The opportunity for support and discussion at the half-day sessions may become increasingly important. The trainee may also find they begin to reject some of their trainer's beliefs and clinical methods and criticise the general running of the practice. These should be regarded as healthy developments.

Management skills

From the start of the year the trainee should have attended practice meetings, but during this phase they should become more interested in how to manage their time, paperwork and patients. The trainee should become involved in all aspects of management from appointment systems to cleaning, from partnership decision making to the ordering of supplies, and can start to make constructive suggestions for improvement.

The trainer will hopefully be enthusiastic, rather than defensive, that the trainee is emerging as a colleague who recognises the need for self-directed learning throughout their professional life, both in clinical and administrative

---

SUMMARY BOX

The partnership phase

The timing will vary with the trainee, but during the second half of the year she or he should make the following changes:

- Increased confidence in the role as a GP
- A balance is struck and the work is no longer viewed as tedious or exciting
- Areas of real difficulty or annoyance are recognised
- Ability to handle distressing or frustrating patients
- Relationship with the trainer becomes less one of dependency, and criticism of the trainer and practice emerge
- Greater interest in how the practice is managed. The trainee will begin to form a view of the kind of practice he would like to work in and how it should be managed.

spheres. A wise trainee will pass through this phase realising their task is not to reorganise the training practice, or change their trainer, but to learn lessons for their future practice. Just as an adolescent learns to leave their family, the trainee should reach the stage when respect for their trainer and training practice remains, but they wish to found their own organisation incorporating their own ideas and practices.

The final phase

The time at the end of the year may appear to pass very quickly. Suddenly the trainee realises there is only a month left and there is still much to be achieved. A planned project is unfinished, visits to other practices have not been made, and gaps in clinical knowledge identified months ago remain. Moreover, this is the time when new commitments have to be considered: sitting the MRCGP, deciding the next job and perhaps moving to a new area.

The trainee will appreciate that all there is to learn about being a GP cannot be taught in a single year and that this is just a 'springboard' for the next stage of learning. They must address how they are to continue to learn after the year is complete; some join a small group of colleagues from the half-day release to study for the MRCGP, others fill educational gaps while doing locum work.

Ending the relationships formed with some patients during the year may be difficult both for the patient and the trainee, and the trainee should give forewarning that they will be leaving. Saying goodbye to the practice team and colleagues at the half-day release course may also be difficult, although contact with the trainer and other members of the practice may continue.

Towards the end of the year the trainee may have become central to the practice and made many friends. Others will not have become so closely

---

SUMMARY BOX

Final phase

In the last month most trainees realise that:

- Not all the objectives identified at the start of the year will be realised
- Time needs to be given to planning what to do after the trainee year has ended
- There is much still to learn and medical training does not end with the year
- Patients should be given forewarning and prepared for their departure
- They must prepare for some sadness at leaving a practice in which they have played an integral part for a year
- The trainee year is but a beginning.

involved but for anybody it is difficult to prepare for their next job while leaving the setting in which they have worked for a year. This departure can be made more difficult by the appointment of a new trainee before the year end, giving the impression that they are being 'pushed out' and are only one in a long line of trainees. The trainee should comfort themselves with the thought that if their year had not been a worthwhile experience, they would not feel sad at its end.

ASSESSMENT

Assessment is essential in any educational programme. Once aims and objectives have been defined, appropriate assessment should be planned to establish whether these are achieved. The nature of assessment affects the knowledge and skills that learners acquire and also their approach to learning. There is at present considerable interest in assessment in general practice, both as a means of monitoring vocational training and as a form of self-audit for established practitioners.

Assessment may be either formative or summative. Formative assessment is designed as part of the educational process, to help learning through feedback, whereas summative assessment (such as an end-point examination) is designed to test attainment at one point in time.

Policies on trainee assessment vary amongst different regions and different trainers. At present the only requirement to proceed from vocational training is a signed certificate of satisfactory completion. The MRCGP examination, though taken by many trainees, is not a requirement for continuing in practice. It does, however, seem likely that in the near future more formalised and compulsory assessment may be introduced for trainees.

It is important that trainers and trainees discuss assessment at the very beginning of the year and reach agreement on a plan for monitoring learning. Ideally the assessment should take place at regular intervals during the year so that progress can be monitored. The main objectives are to identify areas of both strength and weakness in the trainee's learning and ways in which learning can be optimised.

The list below identifies a number of learning methods which can be used for assessment throughout the year:

- Rating scales — where the trainee subjectively rates their confidence and competence in different areas
- MCQs, MEQs, essays and vivas — where an objective assessment of strengths and weaknesses is made
- Learning diary — a diary can focus on the process and outcome of learning
- Checklists
- Case discussions

- Computer programmes, e.g. RCGP Phased Evaluation Project
- Medical record reviews
- Direct observation in surgery
- Observation of video-recorded consultations
- OSCEs (objective structured clinical examinations)
- Trainee project.

SOURCES OF HELP FOR TRAINEES

The trainer

A month into her trainee year, Dr S found she was unhappy with her trainer's approach to training. She become aware of strife between the partners in the practice. Moreover, she found that the brief time she had for tutorials was constantly interrupted and was unstructured. Before she told her trainer that she wanted to leave the practice, she decided to share her problems with him. She was surprised to find how concerned he was. He changed the tutorial time so there were no interruptions, worked with her to draw up a structured programme and took her complaints to a partnership meeting and tried to resolve the partners' conflicts. Within a few weeks she was much happier and remained with the practice.

If a trainer is unable or unwilling to resolve a trainee's problems, the trainee has the option of approaching either the course organiser or the associate advisor for the area.

The course organiser

The course organiser is available to hear the trainee's problems in confidence. They cannot refer these to the trainer without permission from the trainee. This enables the course organiser to support the trainee without any complaint reaching the practice, unless the trainee wishes it to.

The associate advisor

The associate advisor has influence in the reselection of a trainer. They can visit the practice and talk to the trainer about any problems brought to their attention. If no attempt is made by the trainer to address a trainee's problems, this will be considered when the trainer comes up for reselection. If the trainee wishes to leave a practice, the associate advisor can help them find another practice in which to complete the year.

The regional advisor

If problems are still not resolved, the trainee can turn to the Regional Advisor, who is the person ultimately responsible for GP training in their area. With the help of the Regional GP Postgraduate Committee, the trainee can appeal to the Joint Committee for Postgraduate Training in General Practice (JCPTGP) for an additional period of training in another practice.

Dr H did not enjoy a good relationship with his trainer. One or two emergencies were felt to have been mismanaged. The trainer contacted some of the consultants for whom the trainee had previously worked, and found they too were unhappy with his decision making in emergency situations. Towards the end of the year, the trainer informed Dr H that he would not be able to sign the certificate for satisfactory completion of the year (VTR1) on the grounds that he was not competent in handling emergency situations. The trainee discussed this situation with the associate regional advisor and the executive of the GP education committee. A new practice and trainer were found who were prepared to supervise a further 6 months' training. The JCPTGP agreed to fund this additional period. At the end of this time the new trainer signed the VTR1 form.

In most cases, problems can be resolved but sometimes a trainee is not suited to general practice and they do not gain their certificate of satisfactory completion. The obstacle is often not to do with clinical ability but rather their approach to practice.

Dr Y was found by his trainer to be constantly late for his surgeries. Sometimes he missed a whole surgery. He never attended the half-day release course. He missed some tutorials and, when he did attend, came unprepared. He lived a long way from the practice and made no arrangements to find accommodation locally when he was on-call, and instead slept in his car in the practice car park! The trainer also learnt that Dr Y was undertaking private work during the time he should have been in the practice.

Despite the trainer pointing out these shortcomings, Dr Y did not change his habits and eventually was told that unless a significant improvement was made, the certificate of satisfactory completion could not be signed. By the end of the year there had been no change and no certificate was given. A hearing was arranged by a panel of three: the Chairperson of the Education Committee, a different Regional Advisor and a Course Organiser. An appeal went to the JCPTGP for a further 3 months' training in a different practice. Dr Y still failed to improve his approach and he did not receive a final certificate.

Other institutions

During the year, the trainee may find the following organisations of help:

- the BMA (British Medical Association)
- the RCGP (Royal College of General Practitioners)
- the RSM (Royal Society of Medicine)
- the local FHSA (Family Health Service Authority)
- the regional trainee committee
- the Medical Defence or Medical Protection Societies (for medico-legal problems).

Trainees are advised to contact the secretaries of each organisation for further information. Many offer much reduced annual subscriptions to trainees wishing to become members.

There is always the possibility that a patient will take medico-legal action against a doctor or complain to their FHSA. Every trainee should therefore know how to respond in the event of such action, and this is a discussion point for tutorials and the half-day release course.

REGIONAL STRUCTURES CONCERNED WITH TRAINING

The GP Postgraduate Committee

This committee is responsible for GP postgraduate education within the area. Its members include representatives from the trainers' workshops, local medical committees (LMCs), course organisers, RCGP and GP Tutors. The chairperson, along with the Regional Advisor, sits on the Regional Education Board, which controls and funds all postgraduate education. The board is chaired by the Regional Postgraduate Dean. All trainers and course organisers are appointed ultimately by the education committee, although they are interviewed by individual selection committees.

Regional Trainees' Committee

Trainees have their own regional organisation, which comprises a representative from each half-day release course and from each vocational scheme and which meets bi-monthly. This committee has its own chairperson and secretary. It usually arranges an annual regional trainee conference. Each regional committee sends a representative to the national General Medical Council (GMC) Trainee Committee. This national committee organises the annual trainee national conference and manages trainee matters on a national scale. Each regional trainee committee has two representatives on the GP Postgraduate Committee.

The regional administrative structure of GP practice is difficult to grasp at first and the only way to understand it fully is to become involved as a trainee representative. Some trainees find this experience a useful entry into learning about GP politics.

THE HALF-DAY RELEASE SCHEME

Every trainee should attend a half-day release course and needs to attend 80% of its meetings to qualify for the certificate of satisfactory completion. Each scheme is organised by one or two course organisers appointed by the Regional GP Postgraduate Committee. These course organisers have their own regional association, which meets at least twice a year. A National Course Organisers Conference is also held annually.

There are considerable variations in half-day release schemes throughout the UK. In some areas, trainees meet for an entire day, in others, for an extended lunch or afternoon meeting. Most schemes meet throughout the academic term and some include visits, e.g. to a drug treatment unit, AIDS unit, a prison or shelter for the homeless. It is becoming increasingly common for course organisers to include a residential course of 2–3 days, which gives more time for learning and facilitates group cohesion.

The structure and content of schemes are decided by the course organisers, although there will usually be opportunity for the trainees themselves to plan part of the course. The trainees attending come from hospital posts and general practice. In some areas the group members will change throughout the year as trainees are appointed at different times. In others, all trainees join the half-day release at the same time, or at just two points in the year.

Speakers may be invited to talk on a particular clinical subject, e.g. diabetes or AIDS, or on management topics like finance or administration. Time is usually set aside for case discussions. These may be problem cases or patients randomly selected from a recent surgery.

Trainees are encouraged to attend regional trainee courses and the national trainee conference.

STUDY LEAVE

The trainee is entitled to 30 days study leave during the year. Half of this will be taken up attending the half-day release course. The rest will be used to attend training courses or hospital clinics or to visit other practices. At the end of the year, trainees are expected to be able to undertake child health surveillance, practise minor surgery and be competent in resuscitation techniques. Many will want to attend courses in preparation for sitting examinations (see Chs 8 and 9).

Before attending any course, the trainee needs to notify the Regional Advisor's office in order to qualify for reimbursement of the course fees. The trainee should receive a certificate of attendance from the course organiser and this must be sent to their FHSA in order to claim for travel and subsistence expenses. This method of reimbursement also applies for the half-day release residential course.

THE TRAINEE'S RESPONSIBILITIES

As a postgraduate and an adult learner, the trainee is responsible for the organisation of their trainee year. If they are to do this effectively, they must pay particular attention to health and the use of equipment.

Your health

A sick doctor will not give the best care to patients, and is unlikely to enjoy their job. One of the responsibilities of the trainee, like any doctor, is to take care of their own health. They need to register with a GP and subject themselves to the usual screening processes. Also, the trainee must realise that they can fall ill just as patients do, and they should not feel guilty for taking time off for sickness when necessary.

To remain in good health, time away from the practice should be protected and used for family activities, holidays, hobbies, etc. Efficient management of the clinical workload needs to be learnt in order to allow sufficient time away from work. The trainee may also need to learn to be aware of their own feelings and to discuss these with others. Many trainees are surprised by how their emotions are stirred by the situations in which they find themselves as a GP. It is well known that GPs have a high stress level, but they tend to ignore the need to examine their own emotions, which may lead to burnout, alcohol or marital problems. Methods of avoiding stress, depression or sickness should be discussed with the trainer or at the half-day release course and need to be learnt early on in the year.

It is wise for all doctors to be covered by appropriate insurance, and those with dependents should write a will.

Dr J went on holiday to France in the middle of his trainee year and was involved in a road traffic accident. He was badly injured and needed to be flown back to hospital in the UK. As a result he was off work for 6 months. This accident occurred when his wife had given up work to have their second child. The mortgage payment became a problem as he had not insured himself against serious accident. His recovery took place slowly and was filled with financial worries.

Your equipment

Apart from a stethoscope and a car, a trainee is not advised to buy any equipment at the beginning of the year. The training practice is obliged to provide a medical bag and all necessary medical equipment. This should be used by the trainee while they get a feel for different types of equipment. Only when the trainee feels confident in their needs and preferences should they make their own purchases.

Much of the equipment used within the practice is the property of the practice. Trainees should take note of how equipment is used and how it is looked after. They should have hands-on experience during the year of using different equipment, e.g. for taking smears, minor surgery, paediatrics surveillance, examining eyes, performing ECGs, computers, etc.

A few GPs equip themselves to cope with major accidents. For example, GPs in the Hebrides are responsible for dealing with accidents to climbers or fishermen. In many areas organisations such as BASICS (British Association of Immediate Care Schemes) operate a rota to cover major accidents and incidents. These doctors will have undertaken a special course before they invest in resuscitation or other equipment.

All GPs should consider carefully what drugs, dressings and papers they need to carry in their bag or in their car. This will vary from practice to practice and will depend on the number of pharmacies open at night and accessibility of hospital accident and emergency units. Doctors' cars are frequently broken into and medical bags stolen, so insurance cover of all equipment is advised.

Your learning

Everybody learns in a different way. Some do it by reading on their own, while others prefer first to experience a clinical situation and then to read about it. Some enjoy group work, role play or learning from videos. Some benefit from somebody sitting in on their consultations; it makes others feel very uneasy. Doctors may learn through projects, audit, research, teaching or writing, and every trainee must discover which methods of learning best suit them.

A system is needed to identify gaps in learning. Methods include filling in questionnaires, participating in group discussions and attending practice meetings where the relationship is secure enough for doctors to receive and give gentle criticism. A great deal can be learned from listening to the patients, as well as receptionists, nurses, pharmacists and others.

Perhaps the most important skill for the trainee to learn during the year is how to become an effective self-learner. This requires not only learning how to identify and accept areas of ignorance, but also how to deal with them.

YOUR FUTURE

Some trainees have clear ideas about their future plans, either in the short or longer term. The objective of going straight into a partnership after training is no longer so widely held and many doctors prefer to take some time broadening their experience and exploring other avenues. Options include travel and work abroad, further hospital experience, locum work or research and academic posts, which are becoming more popular. One advantage of the trainee year is that it allows time for the trainee to plan a professional future. To do this they must understand the type of doctors they are, what clinical activities they enjoy and what they find difficult. Personal and family situation must obviously be taken into consideration.

For those who intend to seek a partnership soon after training it is important to start looking at possible openings in good time, and to discuss ideas with their trainer and other colleagues. Partnerships are like marriages and most people enter into them with the expectation that it will be a long-term prospect. Do not rush into anything. Try to be clear about the type of practice in which you will be happy working. The main reason why partnerships fail is incompatibility between personalities, so try to gauge how you are likely to get on with potential colleagues.

At the end of their training years, after some time working as locums, Drs K and F became full-time partners in practices in the area where they had trained. Dr K is now a trainer himself. Dr O had a baby shortly after training and later became a job sharing partner in a large group practice. Dr S spent a year in Australia and then became a partner in a rural practice. Dr H entered training in psychiatry. Dr J recovered from his injuries, completed his training and is looking for a post in academic general practice. Dr M did not return to general practice, but continued working as a clinical assistant in ophthalmology and Dr Y is working as a ship's doctor on a passenger liner.

SUMMARY BOX

Points for the trainee to appreciate during the year

- There are many sources of help if the trainee encounters serious problems
- There is a regional structure concerned with training
- The value of the half-day release course and how it is run
- How to obtain and finance study leave
- The trainee is responsible for their:
  — health
  — equipment
  — learning
  — future plans.

2. Health not illness

John Horder

In this chapter I shall explore what has been thought and written about health and about healthy people in order to see how far these ideas are relevant to consultations in general practice and therefore useful to general practitioners and those who now join with them in the work of primary care.

I shall avoid discussion of illness as far as possible. The subject of health has never attracted the attention of doctors to an extent which compares in any way with the attention paid to illness, as a first glance at any medical library will demonstrate. It is comparable to the moments of silence which punctuate many pieces of music or to the spaces which separate objects in a picture.

There are obvious reasons for the inclusion of the subject in this book. One is that the recent National Health Service reforms have emphasised the promotion of health and given prominence to the role of general practitioners in achieving this purpose. It seems therefore logical to reflect on the nature of what is to be promoted and on the characteristics of people who offer the clearest demonstration of it.

A less obvious reason is that doctors themselves, like other people, now inevitably make choices which will affect their own and their families' future health. In the past we have tended to neglect this, at least until something bad happens. Dealing always with ill people it is easy to imagine that illness is something which happens only to others or that ill people expect doctors always to be well, since they depend on them. However, the almost unanimous decision of doctors in this country not to smoke suggests a change of attitude based on sound evidence.

The third and most fundamental reason for including this chapter in a book intended to be a companion to the whole trainee year is that it illustrates the importance of reflecting about what each of us is trying to do when seeing patients or organising a practice. General practitioners have not always had identical aims in their work, although they have often assumed that this is the case and that what they are trying to do is clear enough and beyond any need for discussion. The recent emphasis on audit — reviewing performance — has begun to change this by compelling attention to particular aims before their achievement can be tested.

Perhaps the best-known statement of the aims of medicine is the ancient one:

> To cure sometimes, relieve often, comfort always.

These fine words encapsulate a concern for ill people which does not necessarily stop at combatting a disease. But they do not include either the aim of preventing disease or that of promoting health. The intention in this chapter is to consider health as the ultimate purpose which embraces all these aims. The weight which a particular doctor gives to each of them will still be a personal decision, taken both in relation to each patient and in overall practice policy.

My own interest in the subject arose partly from reflecting on the nature of consultations which I experienced as a general practitioner and partly from reading.

There are many consultations in which patients present problems much as they might take their car to an unknown garage for a fault to be mended. The doctor may respond by some intervention to repair the fault. In most instances it will be mended, whether due to the intervention or to the healing processes of nature. The doctor observes the disappearance of symptoms and signs towards the goal of normality. The patient has relief, as malaise, cough or pain diminish, looks forward to normal activity and may even recognise, by contrast with recent experience, an emerging sense of wellbeing, a sudden awareness of something which has normally been taken for granted and will soon be so again.

But such satisfactorily resolved episodes encourage ideas which will be questioned in this chapter — that health is a person's usual state, that it is sharply distinct from illness; that, when well, body and mind are at their full potential; that most people will be in this state most of the time until old age, except for occasional lapses. These ideas might seem self-evident to younger people, if they describe their own predominant experience. But do they truly reflect reality?

There are, on the other hand, consultations in which repairing a fault seems inadequate or inappropriate because there is a need for something more or different. I have in mind problems which are both more personal and more persistent becoming more apparent to the doctor as he/she sees the same patients repeatedly — people trying to cope with difficulties, whether they arise from their bodies, their minds, their relationship with other people or the environment in which they live. The doctor finds himself or herself increasingly thinking about the person and about the possibilities for supporting or strengthening them. Effective practical interventions may or may not be possible.

A doctor-patient made the need very clear to me on the telephone: 'I don't want you to do anything; I just want you to be there'. Imagine, perhaps, a patient who is born with some congenital disability or who develops multiple sclerosis or who is suffering recurrent depressive states; or perhaps a daughter caring for a parent with Alzheimer's disease — or just some frequent attender who is chronically anxious and consults about one thing after another. I found myself wondering not only about the way in which such problems interfered with the lives people had hoped to lead, but also about what possibility for restoration remained to them. What better state could they achieve, given their circumstances and personalities? Had all hope of health to be abandoned? Were some aspects of healthiness still within reach?

These questions set me wondering about my own aims in trying to help people with such problems. They already went beyond the elimination or alleviation of a disease. They were concerned with achieving a better quality of life, centred around better health. Might it not then be worthwhile to think about the meaning of health, in case something apparently so obvious concealed ideas which could prove unexpectedly useful in practice?

This was ambitious stuff — imprecise, seldom explicit, seldom discussed openly with a patient. But it represented several shifts of focus — from the level of organs or bodily systems to that of a person in an environment, from present to future, from short term to long term, from actual to potential, from the negative aim of trying to eliminate a disease or a harmful influence to the positive one of trying to increase resistance, resilience, ability to cope or sense of wellbeing.

If reading was another influence through which my interest arose, an early example was in the literature about the Peckham Health Centre, an idealistic venture started over fifty years ago in south-east London, with the avowed aim of studying and promoting health in a small community. The venture came to a premature end, partly because of the war and partly through lack of support when the National Health Service started. Its short history left a legacy of interesting observations and pregnant ideas which still make worthwhile reading (Pearse & Crocker 1943).

The Peckham doctors saw their work as an *alternative* to the care of illness, perhaps because they were not in a position to diagnose and treat, but certainly because they believed in the possibility of undermining illness by promoting healthier behaviour.

In this chapter the study and promotion of health is seen as a *complementary* aim. So far from diverting attention from the urgencies of diagnosis, treatment and care, this aim will be perceived as inseparable from them because it is a different but complementary way of thinking about those tasks. Its short title is 'anticipatory care'. This term, by its emphasis on the future consequences of decisions reached in a consultation, makes room for practice in which the care of ill people, the prevention of diseases and the promotion of health form part of the same continuum.

Thus, it is not a question of either/or, but of paying attention to the other side of the same coin, the side which has hitherto been less well illuminated.

Will that side prove to be merely the mirror-image of the study of illness or something distinct?

Why is health important?

It would be ridiculous for anyone to claim that the subject of health is *not* important. Nobody does in fact do so, but this is because any ensuing discussion proves almost always to be about illness. Indeed the work is often used as if it is stood for both health and illness, viz 'National Health Service' or 'ill-health'. I start this exploration not knowing whether I shall be able either to avoid discussing illness or to persuade readers that its neglected opposite is indeed important in itself.

The plan of this chapter

In testing the proposition that the study of health is useful to general practitioners and those who work with them, the first essential is to consider the meaning and nature of health. How then does it relate to illness in people's lives? What are the influences which favour healthiness and how far can they be brought into play by general practitioners?

CONCEPTS AND DESCRIPTIONS OF HEALTH

Everyone knows what health is until they try to describe or define it.

This section displays a variety of ideas about the nature of health derived from several disciplines. How well do they fit together?

There are two preliminary explanations. First, there is no reason to think that health relates only to the body. As with illness, it seems likely to have psychological and social aspects as well as physical ones. Secondly, the word 'illness' is used in this chapter to include both 'disease' — an objective term used by trained people to distinguish one disease from another — and the subjective experience of feeling ill, familiar to trained and untrained people alike.

'A state of complete mental, physical and social wellbeing and not merely the absence of disease or infirmity.' This, the World Health Organization's definition, forms a convenient starting point both because it is well known and because it establishes a fundamental division between negative and positive concepts of health. This makes a convenient way of laying out what follows in this chapter. That said, each half of it is unrealistic in the context of clinical practice, for reasons which are important to discuss below.

1. Health as 'absence of disease or illness'

The concept of health which comes most easily to the mind of people with a medical training is 'the absence of disease' — a state in which no evidence of illness, disease, injury or disability can be found by the well-tried methods of medical enquiry into past and present symptoms, of examination and investigation.

Although negative, this definition is essential and cannot be avoided. It is attractive because it implies a clear line between health and illness which can be identified in any person or group of people. The duty and fascination of detecting and assessing illness leaves most doctors little troubled by its negative form. For people in general, the statement is uninspiring and it puts the topic outside their control, while it remains their concern. Essentially an objective concept, it could have a subjective aspect when a person believes that he or she is without illness.

Before looking at alternatives, it is worthwhile to consider the prevalence, in a population, of health defined in this way. A number of studies make this possible.

Evidence was collected from both the United Kingdom and the United States (White et al 1961), by visiting an unselected sample of people in their homes and questioning them closely about their recent experience of illness, injury or disability, however slight. This showed that, of any 1000 people of 16 years or older, 750 reported having been aware of one or more symptoms in any one month. Thus, by this definition and method, only 25% of a population is healthy. Had symptomless disorders been included, the figure would have been even lower, as it would also have been if the enquiry had covered a period longer than one month.

Absence of disease, injury or disability was also used as one criterion in the rigorous routine examinations repeatedly undertaken for 4000 members of the Peckham Health Centre (all ages) between 1936 and 1950 (Pearse & Crocker 1943). There was a preponderance of younger people. Despite this only 14% of males and 4% of females were found to be without evidence of any disorder, however slight, and therefore healthy by an assessment which did include physical examinations and simple laboratory investigations. Although these people were not complaining or consulting, it could justly be argued that they did not form a random sample of the general population.

If it is also argued that these studies are now out of date, more recent evidence is essentially similar (Wadsworth et al 1971, Bridges-Webb 1974).

One example is from California (Berkman & Breslow 1983). In 1965 a probability sample of 6928 adults completed questionnaires which used four measures (ability to perform certain basic daily activities; presence during the previous year of one or more chronic conditions or impairments; presence during the previous year of one or more symptoms; subjective rating of general energy level): 29% were classified in a no-complaints category, but of this minority not all reported a high energy level.

So, if health is defined negatively as a state in which no evidence of illness, disease, injury or disability can be found, much less than half of any population is completely healthy even during any one month and this figure still varies according to the rigour of the criteria and tests used. Indeed it has even been suggested that a healthy person should be described as someone who has not been fully examined.

2. Health as 'normality'

Closely related to the concept of 'absence of disease' is that of 'normality', whether physiological or psychological. It forms a link between negative and positive concepts of health.

Norms are established 'not only to recognise departures from them in dealing with ill people, but also to provide standards towards which restoration may be directed (Ryle 1947). Since humans are not identical one with another, norms have to be expressed as a range rather than a precise figure. Ryle quotes from the Grant study of 'normal young men' started at Harvard in 1940 (and still continuing), in which examination of 259 subjects showed pulse rates (recumbent) of within the range 40–96 per minute, with a mean of 66.1 and a standard deviation of 10.0. Comparable ranges were recorded for blood pressure, haemoglobin and blood sugar (Heath 1945).

The number of normal physiological or biochemical measurements which might be expected in health is very large. Most relate to particular organs or bodily systems and have been developed in relation to particular diseases. As a test of overall physical capacity a relatively comprehensive single measurement in common use is that of oxygen consumption — the maximal 0^2 uptake attained by an individual during strenuous exertion. The range of normal would, of course, differ for an athlete from that for a bank clerk; and for a young man from that for an older man.

The concept of normality also has a place in psychology or sociology, but a much less secure one. An obvious example is that a normal range is recognised for the intelligence quotient. But when it comes to measurements more relevant to health or illness, the range of normal variation is so wide and so subject to cultural differences as to be of very limited use. It leaves the field open to value judgements and to the exhibition of prejudice. Nevertheless, doctors frequently have to decide when, for example, anxiety or misery has crossed the boundary between normal and abnormal, has become a harmful burden and requires help. Such boundaries are usually definable or measurable only for purposes of a particular piece of research.

General practitioners constantly make rough assessments of normality in history-taking — for instance in recording exercise tolerance, undisturbed sleep of adequate amount, regular menstruation, never smoking, or a family history of longevity. Similarly, physical examination will recognise a heart murmur which is 'innocent' or a hard epigastric lump which proves to be the normal xiphisternum, an occasional cause for considerable anxiety. They monitor the course of normal pregnancy and are increasingly concerned with assessing whether a child's development is normal — an exercise which includes behavioural as well as physical observations. They constantly decide when a patient, after an episode of illness, has returned to normal health and can be signed off.

3. 'Wellbeing'. Positive concepts of health

'It's feeling in your best form, joyful, contented, with a good appetite, sound sleep, a desire to be up and going.' This is one of the many lay descriptions of what it is like to feel healthy, taken from a study in which 80 French people of various ages and social classes were interviewed in depth (Herzlich 1969). Or again: 'I feel alert and can always think of lots to do. No aches and pains — nothing wrong with me and I can go out and jog. I suppose I have more energy. I can get up and do a lot rather than staying in bed and cutting myself off from people'. This quotation is from a similar English study (Blaxter 1990). Or again from France: 'Not being ill certainly — but in addition there is real health — then one's body is used like a well-oiled instrument that one doesn't have to attend to — and it's having eyes that are bright, a good complexion and feeling at ease when one is with friends — not feeling nervous'.

Clearly health as 'wellbeing' is something of which people can be conscious at times, even if it is more often taken for granted and not noticed. In any case, unlike in illness, 'the organs are silent' (Leriche 1936). For some it may be an aspiration rather than an experience at all. The close overlap with other life values, such as happiness or peace of mind, is obvious.

It is also obvious in these quotations that health as wellbeing has physical, psychological and social aspects. The aspect of physical fitness, strength, athletic prowess, is prominent among young people, particularly males. Both sexes talk of a feeling of energy, vitality, enthusiasm for work. 'Health is when I feel I can do anything.' 'Loads of whumph' (Blaxter 1990). The psychosocial aspects are most frequently stressed in this study by women and the better educated. 'I am at peace with myself — energetic, outgoing. I can cope with more pressures than usual, with the demands made by other people. I have the capacity to know when I have had enough, whereas if I am less healthy, tired, I am inclined to go on too long.' 'A joy to be living.' Women in particular are more likely to define health, especially in themselves, in terms of relationships with other people. A young woman: 'I have more patience with my family'. An older woman: 'You're more willing to meet people and help'.

The quotations finally show that health, as wellbeing, entails being able to do things easily, efficiently, quickly — to work hard or long, the ability to cope. 'Being able to do what you want to when you want to.' Even: 'Health is freedom'.

These are descriptions of a cluster of subjective feelings or aspirations. They come close to descriptions of 'ecstasy' (Laski 1980) or 'peak experiences' (Maslow 1968). These are rare, short-lived experiences but never forgotten. Unfortunately they also come close to statements from manic patients or people under the influence of drugs such as heroin. Other features of wellbeing must therefore be considered which link these subjective feelings to values which ensure that they have a reliable and lasting basis.

Genuine wellbeing has a balance of physical, psychological and social aspects (although, as will be seen, it is unrealistic to require that each should be complete). It includes features in each of these categories, but the balance must allow room for the differences between one person and another, even within the same culture — differences such as age, sex, intelligence, education, social class and many others.

The concepts which follow describe features of true wellbeing. They help to explain why some people remain more healthy than others. They can also be seen as aims which doctors and those working with them can help their patients to pursue.

4. Health and wellbeing as physical fitness

Physical fitness is, for some people, an aim in itself and it often induces the positive feelings described. People may achieve exceptional physical strength or skills. There is evidence (Royal College of Physicians of London 1991, Shaper & Wannamathee 1991, Gloag 1992) that physical exercise reduces the risk of certain forms of disease or disability, but not all forms. Some people may be overzealous in this single aim, losing a sense of balance with other aims in life.

For most people fitness means fitness *for* — for whatever roles they are trying to fulfil, but particularly for their work. This will require varying degrees and types of fitness. For the most part people judge for themselves what is required, but for some types of work exacting standards are required and have to be imposed, for instance, for scaffold erectors or for airline pilots. The second example makes it obvious that the concept of fitness does not apply only to the physical aspects of a person. This leads to the wider concept of 'function' or 'functional capacity'.

5. Wellbeing as functional capacity

Function, like physical fitness, is a measurable feature of wellbeing, distinct from the recognition of disease and illness, although it can be linked to this (see WONCA 1990). It offers a clinical approach already familiar to doctors and patients alike as part of what they do every day. It is important for doctors to enquire about people's work and how they cope with it or to ask older people about their mobility or activities in looking after themselves. Questions may need to cover intellectual, emotional or social functions as well as physical, according to the nature and demands of a person's life.

Much of what was discussed earlier under the heading of normality referred to functional capacity, at the levels of both body system and the person.

An accepted definition of function is 'the ability of a person to perform in, adapt to, and cope with, a given environment, measured both objectively and subjectively' (Bentsen 1990). This definition introduces the idea of adaptation into this discussion of wellbeing — a reminder that people inevitably live in an environment and inevitably have to adapt to it as it changes. One of the changes to which they have to adapt is illness.

6. Wellbeing as resistance, resilience or hardiness

The concept of 'resistance' obviously assumes that people exist in an environment and that they may be threatened by influences which diminish health and cause illness. Physically, it is familiar in the form of immunity to infections. This is likely to be associated with physical fitness.

'Resilience' suggests chiefly a psychological characteristic in the face of stress or suffering. As extreme examples, resilience has been studied in air-crew in wartime (Symonds 1970) and in concentration camp victims (Antonovsky et al 1971).

The physical mechanisms of immunity can prevent an infection from taking hold or limit its manifestations. Where, however, physical resistance is incomplete and illness ensues, resilience of mind is challenged as a separate variable. It may succumb or it may overcome.

In this way, health or wellbeing, conceived as resilience, can co-exist with illness or disability. An American author offers the examples of three United States Presidents: Theodore Roosevelt (asthma), Franklin Roosevelt (poliomyelitis) and John Kennedy (chronic back pain). The paradox is discussed later on in this chapter.

The ideas of resistance and resilience are closely related to the idea of health or wellbeing as 'a reserve' — like a store of capital which can be drawn on or replenished when necessary. Like resistance and resilience, health is not equally distributed to everyone, whether because of hereditary endowment or of the circumstances of life or through an individual's own management of this form of capital.

How far do we know the reasons why some people are more resistant or more resilient or have a greater reserve of health than others? Why do some people not break down or become ill, despite severe or continuing stress?

Antonovsky (1980, 1989) has proposed that there are 'general resistance resources'. Unlike the specific immunological response to a particular type of infection (which, for instance, is the basis for one important group of activities in disease prevention), these resources have a wider reference, raising resistance to many different diseases. What are they and how can they be mobilised for people's benefit? Are they accessible to those who work in primary care?

They range from features of the physical environment, such as adequate housing, food, money, appropriate work; to the social environment — the support of spouse, parents, friends and workmates; to personal characteristics, heredity, intelligence, knowledge; to personal attitudes, for example, belief in the possibility of prevention or commitment to a purpose; to personal coping strategies. Physical fitness can, of course, also be seen as a resource increasing resistance and resilience.

Although some of these resources may be outside the control of individuals, even in western countries (e.g. enough money, work and, of course, heredity or intelligence), many are potentially within their control. Some belong to the way in which people see themselves and their world. Several writers have identified attitudes which seem particularly important in explaining why some people subjected to great stress do not get ill or, if ill, do not break down or succumb.

Kobasa et al (1981) see 'hardiness' as made up of three characteristic attitudes: the first is commitment, meaning the ability to believe in the truth, importance and value of what one is doing and of who one is, and therefore to involve oneself — in other words a sense of purpose. The second is 'control — the belief in one's ability to influence the events one experiences (whether alone or in company with others) rather than feeling powerless. 'Hardy' people reject the notion that luck, chance or other more powerful people always determine their fate. People can be broadly divided into those who believe that the 'locus' of control is within themselves and those who believe it is outside themselves. So, for example, 'illness is possibly preventable', versus 'illness is always a matter of fate'.

Kobasa's third characteristic is 'acceptance of challenge' — a belief that change is normal and that it is more likely to be a stimulus or an opportunity than a threat to security. Hardy people are good at tolerating uncertainty.

Here are important personal characteristics — the way in which people see themselves and their world — which a general practitioner may well be aware of in some patients more than others. The question whether they can be influenced or changed is discussed later. Like the personal characteristics of physical fitness, these can be seen as resources for resistance or resilience and so for wellbeing and health.

Antonovksy, pursuing the idea that the way in which people see themselves and their world has a long-term influence on their health comparable in importance to their actual experience of illness, also identifies commitment, sense of control and acceptance of challenge, but adds another important attitude — the conviction that things make sense, are in the main ordered, consistent, clear and not merely random, accidental or unpredictable. The significance of this attitude as a fundamental resource for health and wellbeing is perhaps most obvious in children (Rutter 1985). They need the consistent care and stability which is symbolised by family routines. But stability and routines are important to adults too, alongside the challenge of constant change. They form part of every culture.

It may seem from this discussion of health and resistance, resilience or hardiness that such things as physical fitness have been neglected or that it is unrealistic to give such importance to attitudes of mind alongside the realities of disease, injury and death. But resources such as intelligence, knowledge and belief in prevention do empower some people, both in avoiding encounters with such realities and in using treatment resources wisely.

A HEALTHY PERSON

These ideas about the meaning and nature of health may seem bewilderingly diverse.

Following the World Health Organization's definition, a distinction was made between negative and positive concepts and this has guided the order in which they have been described. The negative concept 'absence of disease or illness' — familiar and unavoidable — came first. Positive wellbeing will have been most obvious in the subjective personal statements quoted, but the concepts of fitness for function, resistance, resilience and even normality all throw light on other aspects of wellbeing. In particular they exclude such semblances of transient wellbeing as can be induced by alcohol or drugs.

It might be expected that all these concepts, each of which is supported by a considerable literature, would be necessary characteristics of healthiness. Should then a healthy person be expected to qualify simultaneously on each and all of the criteria implied?

Dr Richard Asher described 'a case of health' (Asher 1958). His description might seem to fulfil this expectation:

A lady of 90 who was still working. She had worked for 76 consecutive years as a cook and general servant, except for 10 days off with bronchitis when she was 64 and had been nursing her husband in his last fatal illness. She did not consult doctors because she did not believe in them. She was still working from 6.30 am to 10.00 pm at night and cooking for 90 people in a school. She did not leave her post in the holidays. Not surprisingly the headmistress regarded her as a treasure.

Certainly this lady seems to have combined near-freedom from disease (and so resistance and resilience) with fitness for function, a balance between autonomy (attitude to doctors) and interdependence (in the school and her work, which she never left). But the available information is limited. Many questions could still be asked, for instance about minor illness, injury, disability: about childhood and about childbirth: about fulfilment in a life apparently confined to working. Even her single admitted illness and her bereavement remind one that complete wellbeing and absolute freedom from illness are too much to expect.

Reality is more complex. Absence of disease or illness, as argued earlier, is rare even over short periods of time. So is the sense of wellbeing as described. If these terms are understood to cover psychological and social as well as physical experience — as they must be — the difficulty is multiplied. For example, a study of apparently healthy graduate students in California concluded: 'The luckiest of the lives here studied had its full share of difficulties and private despair ... The conclusion to which the study has come is that pathology is always with us.' (Barron, 1963).

Reality is not well represented by any definition of health which implies that health and illness are mutually exclusive or that either must be complete. Unfortunately this applies to the World Health Organization's definition.

SYNTHESIS OF THE CONCEPTS

Health is a complex idea that stands for a range of welcome experiences which people can also recognise in the experience of others. At the same time it stands for subsidiary concepts proposing qualities which can be observed either in a person or group of people. These are proposed by different observers, from the thinking and language of their discipline, but they can all be seen as aspects of one basic idea.

'Health' is always shadowed by 'illness', which is an equally complex idea, although more familiar to doctors or nurses.

People inevitably live in an environment. This is the reality to which concepts of health or illness must relate or within which they may relate to each other. The environment is understood here to include both the physical and social milieux in which people live. They are always changing and people have to adapt to the changes in some way. They may adapt successfully or fail to do so.

Alongside inevitable engagements with the external environment, individuals also have to adapt to such changes within themselves as birth, growth, ageing and the self-generated demands experienced as a result of having a measure of free will.

Changes in the external or internal environment prove beneficial or harmful depending on their nature, extent, timing or relation to other changes. This is so whether one considers the content of the air breathed, the behaviour of other people or the demands made by oneself or others upon one's capabilities.

Health can now be seen as a person's successful adaptation to his or her environment. Fitness for function or for role can be seen as a particular form of adaptation (roles are inevitable in a family, workplace or larger society). Resistance or resilience are qualities of a person faced with environmental challenges which are sensed as threatening or harmful, among them disease or injury. Such a person will seek to prevent trouble before it comes, to cope with it energetically or to accept it if it is inevitable or irreparable. The subjective sense of wellbeing can be seen as a consequence of successful adaptation.

It is not necessary to require that health is achieved only when *all* criteria are fulfilled with all the concepts in evidence simultaneously.

Are illness and disease then always evidence of failure of adaptation within the external or internal environment? They can equally reasonably be seen as evidence only of engagement with some influence for harm or for change. The outcome of the engagement may be unfavourable or favourable. Fever is an example. Infections sometimes kill, but they more often heighten resistance, sometimes for life. The experience of illness or disability endured can diminish resilience but it can also heighten it. Successful adaptation to illness can make people more mature or more considerate to others. Some illnesses seem to play a truly valuable part in a person's life.

THE RELATION BETWEEN HEALTH AND ILLNESS

Must not a satisfactory definition of health allow for the following observations: first, that there are degrees of health as there are of illness; secondly, that the two states cannot be clearly demarcated from each other, either in individuals or populations? A person can fulfil many or all the criteria described here while living with a disability, injury or disease. He or she can even adapt to feeling ill, showing resistance and resilience and other qualities described here.

Thus a diagrammatic view of the relation between health and illness would have to show first a continuum between two poles, without any point of demarcation. Not either/or, but more of one, less of the other. Any individual might find him or herself at different points on the continuum at different times, since people go through bad patches and usually come out of them again. Some people — a minority well known to general practitioners — seem always to vary round a lower position than the majority; their life-long experience and best potential seem to be located always near the illness end of the range. Another less obvious minority seems always to be nearer to the healthy end.

But the diagram of a single continuum would not in itself allow for the evidence already provided that degrees of illness or disease do not necessarily control a person's degree of wellbeing. The two are not completely correlated (Fig. 2.1).

It may seem paradoxical that health and illness can co-exist and are not mutually exclusive alternatives. But this is common experience. For example, members of the Peckham community referred to above were questioned in a way which allowed them to comment on their subjective states. Despite the objective evidence that the majority of the group had some symptom or sign of illness, two out of three said that they felt quite well. 'In my usual health.' 'My health is excellent despite my disability.' Cartwright et al (1973) quotes: 'a daughter reported that her mother "had

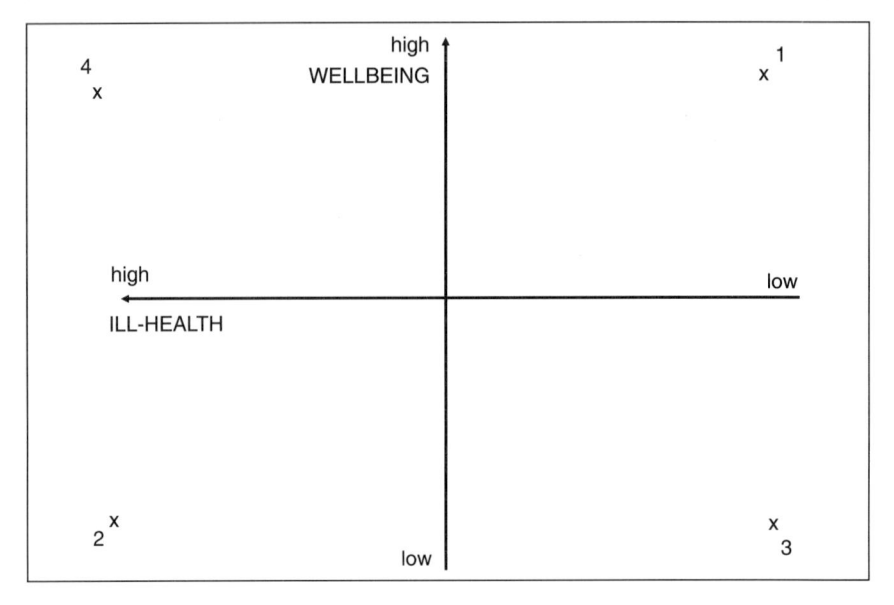

```
                    high ↑
    4              WELLBEING              1
    x                                     x



    high                                  low
    ◄─────────────────────┼─────────────────►
    ILL-HEALTH



         x                              x
    2                                      3
                     low
```

Fig. 2.1 The relationship between wellbeing and ill-health. Of four individuals (numbered 1–4), the first is free of illness and has a high level of wellbeing. The fourth has a high level of wellbeing despite a high level of illness. (Adapted with permission from Downie et al 1990.)

been an active woman before this, with no previous restriction apart from general old age, deafness, loss of sight in one eye and loss of memory"'. Most people have a prejudice for describing their health as being good or at least 'as good as possible'. Exceptions are found chiefly among single-handed parents, the unemployed and people living in industrial areas. People are also less optimistic who show personality characteristics such as neuroticism, as measured by the Eysenk Personality Inventory (Blaxter 1990).

There are interesting studies of:

1. patients on a general practitioner's list who attend less than once in ten years, compared with those who attend at least once a year (Kessel & Shepherd 1965);
2. men working in an oil refinery who had not had a day's absence through sickness over eight years, compared with frequent absentees (Taylor 1968).

In both studies, the incidence of minor illness was the same in the contrasted groups, but there was a slight advantage to the index groups in their experience of more serious troubles. However, many of the rare absentees from work had abnormalities on physical examination at the time of interview. What stands out and impressed the authors in both studies is the difference in attitude to illness between the groups. The non-consulters in the first study took a more favourable view of their own health in the past, present and future than the majority and worried less about it (they were not found to have consulted elsewhere). Those rarely absent from industry differed from their colleagues by denying that there was anything wrong with their health (or with their work or their home). They were almost unanimous in saying that they enjoyed their work. 'Staying away from work or return to work does not depend upon the start or the cessation of a particular disease process, but on the standard of health which the patient sets himself.' (Chieseman, 1959).

It is because of such evidence that health can fairly be seen as 'a way of reacting to problems, not the absence of them' (Barron, 1963). Although it is tempting to dismiss these attitudes as mere optimism in the face of objectively measurable disease, the patient's estimates deserve to be taken seriously. Overall self-estimates of healthiness ('Is your health good, fair, poor, compared with someone of your own age?') prove to be among the best available predictors of mortality (Singer et al 1976) as well as an important aspect of adjustment to major illness (Hunt et al 1980). For general practitioners and others involved continuously with ill people, some of whom must live with their problems, it seems a useful understanding, thus health is:

'A state of *optimal* physical, mental and social wellbeing and not merely a *low incidence* of disease or infirmity.'

THE CONCEPTS APPLIED — THE CONSULTATION

This chapter, so far, has dealt mainly with abstract, general concepts which aim to display the meaning and nature of health. Their application in the consultation now has to be considered.

The consultation in general practice deals with particulars, each case differing from the one before or the one after. The variety and disconnectedness in a morning's work would be one of the first things to strike any new observer, who might well be excused for seeing the overall aim as one of restoring order out of chaos.

The same consultation is likely to look different to different observers according to their background, training and interest. (They will mainly see what relates to what they already know.) Despite a common training, this is also true for doctors. Different doctors do not notice exactly the same points or think about them in exactly the same way. When they conduct consultations, their aims will not necessarily be identical, even for the same case.

This chapter is concerned with a way of thinking about consultations which might influence their conduct. It emphasises the patient's future and the objectives to be pursued by the doctor, the patient or both. It seeks to relate objectives to the general aim of increasing health and to promote a form of practice in which the care of ill people, the prevention of diseases and the promotion of health are parts of the same continuum.

Current practice most commonly relates objectives to the general aim of eliminating or preventing diseases.

There is nothing incompatible about these two general aims. Indeed, there are many consultations in which they are like the two sides of the same coin. For example, faced by a child with tonsillitis, most doctors would not only think of ways of eliminating infection or relieving pain, but also think ahead, if only to establish a time after which progress should be checked. Likely improvement by that time would be pictured.

Taking a more serious condition as an example — coronary occlusion in a 50-year-old male — obviously the preservation of life and the relief of pain are the first objectives. But there are also future concerns: to prevent complications, to preserve or restore normal cardiac function, to restore the patient to normal working life if possible or to plan a more appropriate one if necessary. Care will also need to take into account the reaction of a person and a family to a life-threatening illness which could recur. The need not only for future medical supervision but for possible changes in attitudes and habits will have to be considered. Returning to concepts of health, self-confidence, autonomy, control and resilience become important issues. Resources for health — such as the support of family, friends and workmates, or the patient's understanding of the illness, belief in the possibility of influencing his own future, commitment and will to live — are worthwhile considerations which a doctor can sometimes influence. Querido (1959) showed how such apparently peripheral considerations have a very significant influence even on the final outcome of surgical interventions.

Has this approach anything to offer in cases where deterioration and death are inevitable, for instance multiple sclerosis or terminal cancer? Here, obviously, is the starkest challenge to the possibility of health or the fulfilment of a person's potential. Resistance in the immunological sense fails. Control of self and the person's own world slips away. Is there any sense in which wellbeing as resilience is possible? For some, faith in a future life is real, but not for all. For most, the time remaining and capacities retained become more precious and close relationships can grow richer, but not for all. As in less serious life crises, acceptance — coming to terms with the inevitable — is achieved by many people. Some, given the chance, will choose to talk about such painful issues with the doctor or nurse who is willing, above all, to listen and give time, without evasion. Such help in such circumstances can prove valuable beyond all expectation.

Nothing has been described in these examples which cannot be found in the best contemporary practice, but these considerations are easily neglected if practice is concentrated on a reaction to immediate events without forethought, or confined to thinking about issues of disease.

General practitioners, especially when they are established in a locality, deal with many patients who consult about a variety of diseases at the same or different times. They are also consulted about problems in people's lives which can be labelled 'disease' only with difficulty or not at all. The focus of their concern in both instances will have moved towards a familiar person in his own environment. There may nevertheless be choices to be made, by patient or doctor, which will influence their future health.

A common example is the reaction to loss of a spouse or a loved parent. This could probably be called a reactive depression, but it is certainly not a disease. The way this crisis is coped with can have a profound effect on a person's future. Some people are not the same again: some die soon after, unexpectedly. A few commit suicide. Parkes & Weiss (1983) have provided convincing evidence that skilled and trusted support can influence the ultimate outcome, essentially by helping the bereaved person to face reality and to 'give up' (in the sense of relinquish).

There is a minority of people in every practice who are frequent attenders. Among them will be a small number for whose frequent attendance there seems to be no obvious, rational or single explanation. They can be frustrating as well as puzzling. They take up time, but change little. Some seem to put the doctor into a corner where he is without resource and feels the pain of failure. The hostility in a few is thinly veiled or overt. The generic term 'heart-sink' patients (O'Dowd 1988) has a poignant meaning for most of us, but in reality what these people have in common is less important than their individual characteristics and problems. Like people with incurable disease, these people offer the hardest challenge to concepts of health; are such concepts still of any help to doctor or patient?

My own experience in such cases has been of a few successes and many seeming failures. Even the successes have often been extremely limited. Yet there has been a fascination about these challenges, and small successes have brought a reward in satisfaction at least equal to that of achieving much greater benefit for others much more easily.

Such patients are hopeless and helpless in so many different ways that any one example must have limited value. But I think first of a 50-year-old down-and-out who was persistently hostile. His first consultation, with an excellent trainee, ended with him overturning her desk. He became my responsibility. Everything I did was wrong, but he was a frequent attender despite this. Within weeks a major crisis arose when he enriched all the health centre's lavatories with expletives in indelible red letters. My partners, knowing by now that this man had excluded himself from every shelter in London by similar behaviour, offered him one more chance, but only one. The effect was dramatic. He changed from then on to a loyalty in which one doctor and one nurse among us became his trusted friends. Of course we still had to go on tolerating his aggressive ways at times, but he was no longer impossible. He died of cancer five years later. The two of us were the only attenders at his burial and I inherited his only legacy, a paper bag containing a crucifix. He was the son of a prostitute and had never known a father.

This extreme example relates negatively to all the concepts of health. This man experienced serious disease, notably bronchitis and carcinoma of the lung. He smoked heavily. He had been unemployable for years. His behaviour created his world, in which there was no sense of control of events, no self-esteem; no feeling that the world made sense, was consistent or predictable. The only time he had known some sort of wellbeing was when he lived with a woman so full of phobias that she could not go out, so that he had to do everything for her. To this extent he had had for a time a worthwhile purpose in life and had shown 'the capacity to love and work' — Sigmund Freud's definition of health.

THE GENERAL PRACTITIONER AS A RESOURCE FOR PROMOTING HEALTH

In all these examples, a general practitioner and those who work with him or her are dealing with a life which will continue and, of course, with a person. Few people present difficulties like those in the last example, but many have problems which continue or recur or are linked to a different problem in the past or present or in their family; the doctor is aware of these problems. The relevance to whatever problems they present of their personal beliefs, attitudes, knowledge, self-understanding or behaviour can become obvious if a doctor pays attention and gets to know them. The characteristics of general practice offer linked opportunities for recognising their relevance and sometimes for helping a person to change and to reach a little nearer to their best potential.

It is possible to conduct a practice without developing these insights — by concentrating entirely on the effective management of diseases. But this is not in the best tradition of personal care in this country — a tradition which is always under threat, whether, for example, from failure of continuity or communication within group practices, or from the introduction of alien principles by outsiders, or simply from the difficulties of managing time.

Nothing in this chapter diminishes the importance of preventing, curing or relieving specific diseases or of thinking in terms of pathology. Its purpose is to balance those aims with the reminder that people also have other needs, in which doctors and nurses can help them.

Earlier in this chapter, the idea of 'general resistance resources' (Antonovksy 1980) was described and some examples were listed. It was proposed that such resources have a wide reference, raising resistance to a variety of diseases and differing in this way from specific resources for preventing particular diseases, such as immunisation against diphtheria.

Specific resources for prevention are the subject of the next chapter in this book. The question at this point in the present discussion is how far the general practitioner or members of the primary care team can employ these more general resources in order to increase the resistance or resilience of a patient, family or even the population of a practice.

These resources can be classified in the present context as material, social and personal. Money is the most obvious material resource. General practitioners are empowered to write certificates which provide money. Without these, the resistance of the poorer members of the community would be reduced. Social support includes personal services which doctors can mobilise to help elderly people living at home, to relieve carers or to support the mentally ill. Without these, their resistance and resilience would be reduced. More intimately, doctors can influence the attitude of close family members, for example, in understanding the nature of a depressive illness or of phobias. Personal resilience in the face of chronic or recurrent illness depends to some extent on intelligence and knowledge — whether in learning about the illness, learning how to control its manifestation or how best to use available services. These are resources which doctors and nurses can help people to obtain. They can also influence emotional resilience by encouraging the exhibition of feeling or helping to restore self-respect. In dealing with small children, older children or adolescents, there are fundamental and lasting opportunities for helping parents to understand the needs of the young. At the physical level, the value of exercise as a general resource for raising resistance to a number of disorders is well documented; so is the value of not smoking and of drinking in moderation. Neither of these is specific to a single disease.

Here then, are a few examples of opportunities for those who work in primary care to think and act in terms of health. Many of them put the professional in the role of teacher, facilitator, encourager or listener, because changes are bought about only by the patient.

The basic responsibility for health lies with each individual. For the most part, people can be influenced to act or to change only if they see good reason. The skill of doctor or nurse must then be in bringing them to this point if they believe that change would be beneficial. Exhortation is seldom effective. Negotiation is more likely to succeed, but success is particularly associated with teamwork or influence from more than one source simultaneously; also if there is community participation in personal changes (Stott 1986).

Doctors or nurses are, of course, significant providers of social support, especially for those who have few or no others to turn to. Certain familiar principles of behaviour deserve to be recalled. People trust and feel safe with a doctor or a nurse if they feel both understood and valued; the ways in which they are received, kept waiting, summoned, recognised and greeted, all have much more influence on how they feel themselves valued than such trivialities might suggest. Whether they feel understood depends on their reception, that they are allowed to talk, that the doctor both listens and hears and shows obvious interest and accepts what is offered without critical comment or personal rejection. This particularly applies to patients whose self-esteem, for whatever reason, is low or who feel that they are personal failures.

Self-esteem is always at risk in the young, the very old, and in those disabled in body or mind through past or chronic illness. Their particular needs differ, but the doctor or nurse whose knowledge and experience allows them to anticipate needs broadly and identify them exactly is likely to be a source of great strength.

One study must suffice to underwrite the claims of this chapter. A Dutch study of 1500 women and their 75 general practitioners points to a better subjective sense of health (and to a lesser extent better objective health) among patients of family doctors who were observed to offer a style of practice characterised by maximum scores on patient and goal-oriented approaches. These doctors perform many necessary, but few superfluous, diagnostic activities, keeping to a minimum number of referrals and a minimum number of prescriptions for non-specifc medicines. Compared with the patients of other doctors whose style was more interventionist, the patients of these doctors had more realistic expectations about the possibilities for self-care versus professional medical care for common ailments and they visited the doctor less frequently. As patients usually spend many years on the personal list of a general practitioner in the Netherlands, it seems most probable that general practitioners educated their patients during the many consultations which they had with them over this period (Huygen et al 1992).

CONCLUSION

This chapter has sought to throw light on 'health' because it is the overall objective of all the decisions and actions taken by doctors, nurses and those other professionals who work alongside them to help patients and carers. In accepting the now traditional coupling of wellbeing with the relative absence of disease or illness, it has sought particularly to throw light on wellbeing, because this is less likely to be familiar to readers. It has shown a state which often passes unnoticed, but which sometimes becomes a conscious experience which can be described. The experience permeates thoughts, feelings, relationships and behaviour. Although different people emphasise different aspects, they all talk of something desirable. Their descriptions have sufficient in common such that they can be generalised into concepts, through which we might hope to identify positive qualities and aims which contribute to health. These may give a clearer indication of the routes leading to it and so guide efforts in health promotion. These concepts direct attention to improving physical stamina and resistance, to encouraging resilience and other qualities which help people to cope not only with illness or disease but with many other problems in life.

The second part of the chapter seeks to show possible applications of these concepts within the most essential element in primary care — the consultation. In emphasising the individual person, the person's future and the person's potential for health, it argues that health, as illuminated by the concepts, is not completely incompatible with the presence of illness or disease. A disabled or an ill person is not totally divorced from every aspect of wellbeing.

Emphasis on the consultation with individuals has entailed neglect of the health of populations. In this country even general practice has its identifiable population. The concepts discussed are just as relevant in that context, but their application in this way has not been illustrated. It must suffice to point out that health promotion is most effective when its message reaches an individual by more than one route.

Another regretted omission is about the relationship between health and length of life; such evidence as can be found suggests that the relationship is less close than common sense might suggest.

The close relationship between health and happiness is likely to have been obvious to any reader of this chapter. The chapter has dealt with health as a major aim in the life of every person. It is perhaps worth a reminder that it must also be seen as a means towards achieving other fundamental aims.

Look to your health, and if you have it, praise God and value it next to a good conscience as the *second* blessing that we mortals are capable of.
Walton Izaak, 1653. *The Compleat Angler*

At the beginning of the chapter two questions were put. How far are these ideas relevant to consultations in general practice and how far are they useful? The reader will wish to judge for himself or herself.

ACKNOWLEDGEMENTS

I am grateful, for their comments, to Dr Alexis Brook, Mrs Ruth Brook, Professor Avedis Donabedian, Professor Margot Jefferys, Lady J. Medawar, Dr Julian Tudor Hart and my wife, Dr Elizabeth Horder; to Doreen Dahl, my secretary for her careful work, and to Dr Christopher Donovan who first stirred my interest in the subject of this chapter.

REFERENCES

Asher R 1958 A case of health. British Medical Journal 1: 393
Antonovsky A 1980 Health, stress and coping. Jossey-Bass, San Francisco
Antonovsky A, 1989 Unravelling the mystery of health. How people manage stress and stay well. (Social and behavioural science series.) Jossey Bass, San Francisco
Antonovsky A et al 1971 Twenty-five years later: a limited study of the sequelae of concentration camp experience. Social Psychiatry 6: 186–193
Barron F 1963 Personal soundness in university graduate students. In: Creativity and psychological health. D van Nostrand, Princeton
Bentsen B G 1990 The history of health status assessment from the point of view of the general practitioner. In: Functional status management in primary care. Springer Verlag, New York
Berkman L F, Breslow L 1983 Health and ways of living. The Alameda County Study. Oxford University Press, New York.
Blaxter M 1990 Health and lifestyles. Tavistock Routledge, London
Bridges-Webb C 1974 The Traralgon health and illness survey. Part II: Prevalence of illness and use of health care. International Journal of Epidemiology 3: 37–45

Cartwright A, Andersen R 1981. General practice re-visited. Tavistock, London
Cartwright A, Hockey L, Anderson J L 1973 Life before death. Routledge Kegan Paul, London
Chieseman W E 1959 Clinical aspects of absenteeism. The Royal Society of Health Journal 77: 681–686
Downie R S, Fyfe C, Tannahill A 1990 Health promotion, models and values. Oxford University Press, Oxford
Gloag D 1992 Exercise, fitness and health. Editorial. British Medical Journal 305: 377-378
Heath C W 1945 What people are. A study of normal young men. Harvard University Press, Cambridge, Mass
Herzlich C 1969 Santé et Maladie. Mouton, Paris
Hunt S M, McKenna S P, McEwan J, Backett E M, Williams J, Bapp E 1980 A quantitative approach to perceived health status: A validation study. Journal of Epidemiology and Community Health 34: 281–286
Huygen F J A, Mokkink H G A, Smits A J A, Van Son J A J, Meyboom W A, Van Eyk J Th 1992 Relationship between the working styles of general practitioners and the health status of their patients. British Journal of General Practice 42: 141–144
Kessel N, Shepherd M 1965 The health and attitudes of people who seldom consult a doctor. Medical Care (UK) 3: 6
Kobasa S C, Maddi S R, Courington S 1981 Personality and constitution as mediators in the stress-illness relationship. Journal of Health and Social Behaviour 22: 368–378
Laski M 1980 Everyday ecstasy. Thames & Hudson, London
Leriche R 1936 De la santé à la maladie. Encyclopédie Française 6. 16. 1
Maslow A H 1968 Towards a psychology of being. 2nd edn. Van Nostrand Reinhold, New York
O'Dowd T C 1988 Five years of heart-sink in general practice. British Medical Journal 297: 528–530
Parkes C M, Weiss W 1983 Recovering from bereavement. Basic Books, New York
Pearse I H, Crocker L H 1943 The Peckham Experiment. A study of the living structure of society. Allen & Unwin, London (reprinted 1985 Scottish Academic Press, Edinburgh)
Querido A 1959 Forecast and Follow-up. An investigation into the clinical, social and mental factors determining the results of hospital treatment. British Journal of Preventive and Social Medicine 13: 33–47
Royal College of Physicians of London 1991 Medical aspects of exercise; benefits and risks. Royal College of Physicians, London
Rutter M 1985 Resilience in the face of adversity. Protective factors and resistance to psychiatric disorder. British Journal of Psychiatry 147: 589–611
Ryle J A 1947 The meaning of normal. Lancet 1: 1–4
Shaper A G, Wannamathee G 1991 Physical activity and ischaemic heart disease in middle-aged British men. British Heart Journal 66: 384–394
Singer E, Garfinkel R, Cohen S M. Srole L 1976 Mortality and mental health. Evidence from the mid-town Manhattan restudy. Social Science and Medicine 10 (11–12); 517–525
Stott N C H 1986 The role of health promotion in primary health care. Health Promotion 1:49–53
Symonds C 1970 The human response to flying stress. In: Studies in neurology. Oxford University Press, London, 250–270
Taylor P 1968 A study of 194 men with contrasting sickness absence experience in a refinery population. British Journal of Industrial Medicine 25: 106–118
Vaillant G E 1979 Natural history of male psychologic health. New England Journal of Medicine 301: 1249–1254
Wadsworth M E J, Butterfield W J H, Blaney R 1971 Health and sickness. The choice of treatment—perception of illness and use of services in an urban community. Tavistock Publications, London.
White K L, Williams T F Greenberg B G 1961 The ecology of medical care. New England Journal of Medicine 265: 885–892
W O N C A (World Organisation of National Colleges and Associations of General Practice) 1990 Functional status of measurement in primary care, Springer Verlag, New York

SECTION 2

In practice

3. Behind the scenes — how general practice is organised

Steve Brant

INTRODUCTION

Why should a trainee read this section? There is so much else to learn in the year. However, at the end of this time, the trainee will be hunting for a job and looking for clues as to where to work over the years ahead. An assessment of the organisation of a practice and its personnel, including the doctors, will provide much essential information for this task.

Setting out the details of how general practice is organised and how individual practices run does not explain the diversity and individuality of the profession. Each point of organisation raises as many questions as it answers. Why do some GPs practise from modern purpose-built premises and others from small surgeries over a parade of shops? Why do some GPs prefer to work single-handed whilst others practise in groups of ten or more? Why do some GPs use deputising services when others prefer to do all their own out-of-hours calls? It may be that there is no right or wrong answer to these questions but rather an individual solution appropriate to the individuals concerned at that particular time and place. If a standard service is sought then you might expect similar organisational features in much the same way that other services operate — for example, note the similarity in the way departmental stores function in this country. Perhaps the apparent differences in general practice organisation are just that — illusory or superficial with common threads underneath once the surface differences are peeled away.

The trainee is no longer expected to be a passive subject but can use her or his initiative and personality in the service of the patient. The organisation of the practice will shape this development and influence the way the trainee practises for the rest of his/her career. Furthermore, the presence of the trainee may have a direct effect upon the organisation of the practice itself. There is not necessarily a right or a wrong way to organise a practice, and the way that it is run may be seen as an expression of the individuals concerned. Consequently the trainee year provides a unique first-hand opportunity for trainees to decide what sort of practice they would like to work in as principals. It may also demonstrate some of the difficulties of introducing change into an established organisation.

This chapter will explore some of these issues by sketching an outline of the structure of general practice and then looking at some of the advantages and disadvantages contained within it. At the end of this chapter, the trainee will have more idea of the options available and how these may affect practice job satisfaction as well as remuneration. The comments and ideas in this chapter may be provocative and lead to debate. Further reading will be suggested for those who want to explore this area of general practice.

DISCUSSION POINT

Essential equipment? Desks

It is generally now thought that, for optimal communication to take place between GP and patient, they should sit at an angle across the corner of the desk Fig. 3.1).

Patient	
	Desk
	Doctor

What is the evidence that this is the case?
— Are there any circumstances in which this does not apply?
— Why do you need a desk at all — there are some GPs who have dispensed with them and both doctor and patient sit in comfortable armchairs?

I. THE CONTRACT

General practice is organised in such a way that a service can be provided and paid for. From 1965 until 1990 GPs had been working under the Family Doctor Charter which was agreed between the profession and the Government. In April 1990 a new contract (Department of Health 1989) was introduced against the wishes of a large number of doctors.

There were two main intentions of these changes. The first was to make doctors directly accountable for the costs of providing a comprehensive health care service. The second was to improve this service by setting targets, e.g. for child immunisation, and by regular monitoring of particular groups of patients.

The main requirements of the 1990 GP Contract are set out in Table 3.1.

Table 3.1 Main requirements of the 1990 GP Contract (Department of Health 1989)

A. Doctors should render services to patients accepted on to their lists to include:
Health advice
Consultations
Vaccinations
Referrals

B. Additionally they may provide:
Contraceptive services
Child health surveillance
Minor surgery
Maternity medical services

C. Consultations for screening should be offered to:
New patients
Those patients not seen within three years
Yearly to patients aged 75 and older

D. GPs are required to:
Keep adequate records
Issue prescriptions
Prepare practice leaflets
Prepare annual reports

Each part of the contract imposes obligations on the doctor. These require different skills, organisational as well as clinical, to be carried out satisfactorily. Some tasks can be delegated, whereas others must be carried out by the doctor. There is debate over the medical value of some parts of the contract which may require considerable resources to be fulfilled. This needs to be looked at carefully.

A. Personal medical services

Consulting

The terms of service require that, for patients accepted on the list of the doctors, the doctor shall render all necessary and appropriate personal medical services of the type usually provided by general medical practitioners. This includes offering to patients consultations and, where appropriate, physical examinations and arranging for the referral of patients as appropriate for the provision of any other services.

Surgeries

The principal obligation on GPs is to be available to see their patients either at the practice premises or by visiting them at their home. Sometimes it may be necessary to see patients elsewhere, for example, at a local cottage hospital, but most people will be seen at the practice premises.

A busy large group practice may have 200 or more patients attending every day. Consequently, a major constraint upon general practitioners is the amount of time available to fulfil their commitments. Practice organisation is therefore largely based upon efficient use of time.

Most practices have now adopted appointment systems for consultations in the belief that there is less time wasted, but this may not always be coincident with the wishes and desires of the patients. Thus there are still a number of complaints from patients about difficulty in getting to see or speak to their doctor or about delay in getting a doctor to visit.

The principal advantage of an appointments system is that control of access of patients to the surgery is obtained, allowing for a steady stream of work, preventing overcrowding in the surgery and providing a reasonable amount of time for each patient. If the doctors keep to the appointment times, then there is a limited period of waiting for each patient to be seen. Thus the workload can be planned ahead and patients know that when they come to the surgery, they will not have long to wait. The converse of this is that if the appointments are fully booked, the patients may have a delay in being able to see the doctor of their choice and that if the appointment times are not kept surgeries may run very late. It is not reasonable to expect a patient to wait over an hour after his or her appointment time. The responsibility for this delay is the *doctor's*.

Efficient use of time involves surgeries starting and finishing on time. This means that doctors need to be able to terminate consultations and handle telephone interruptions without appearing rude or reducing their clinical effectiveness. This can be quite difficult to do and GPs have developed different methods of handling these situations, such as showing the patient to the door while still talking (Pendleton 1985)!

Someone attending a non-appointments surgery may expect to have to wait. However, if an appointment has been made, perhaps requiring time off work, then if there is a long delay and, subsequently, perhaps only a short time spent in the surgery, this can lead to considerable patient dissatisfaction.

Advantages of a non-appointments surgery are that a person knows that if they attend a surgery, they will be able to be seen by a doctor, even if this means they will have to wait. For the doctor, it means that there will be as much or as little work to do as demand dictates, and thus if very few people attend, they will be able to get on with paperwork or other work as necessary. The disadvantage of this system is that it is impossible to plan what the workload will be. It may vary enormously and if a non-appointment surgery is very busy, the patients may have a very long time to wait. The waiting room may become extremely full, putting pressure on everybody concerned.

In view of these relative advantages and disadvantages, often a mixture of the two systems may be adopted, with the majority of consultations using an appointment system and a period of time being set aside for emergencies every day on a first-come, first-served basis.

Effective use of time entails compartmentalisation, specialisation of various partners into their particular interests, for example minor surgery, and delegation, so that more responsibilities are devolved to other members of the staff, e.g. the practice nurse. If this is done then more time is available for seeing patients with particular needs.

Telephone calls Another form of consulting is by telephone. As most people now have telephones, more time is spent by doctors in this particular method of communication. The number of direct face-to-face consultations has remained relatively constant or slowly dropping over the last few years, and is now at about 3.1 consultations per patient per annum. The number of telephone consultations has been rising considerably and now accounts for about 5% of GPs' workload in the United Kingdom.

The rest of the time in the surgery is devoted to administrative matters such as writing letters and repeat prescriptions, reading mail and communicating with other members of the primary health care team and hospital colleagues. Time also needs to be made available to check immunisation status of children and cervical cytology status of women.

Home visits Home visits are traditionally a characteristic of the British way of general practice. This tradition does not exist in the United States, where virtually all patients who do not attend a surgery go to hospital. This may be partly due to different attitudes to illness and disease but may reflect the different organisation of health care provision in the USA where most of the cost may be borne by the patient.

In the United Kingdom it is believed that visiting patients in their own home offers a unique opportunity to visualise their own particular social, psychological and emotional situations in a holistic approach, offering a better guide to the most likely way the GP may provide assistance and support. However, this may not be a cost-effective approach because it is only possible to visit 2 or 3 patients per hour. In the surgery 6–10 patients may be seen in the same time.

Home visits may either be new requests because of acute problems or the regular monitoring of housebound people for more chronic situations, such as the elderly with cardiac failure on regular medication. The number of such visits has fallen in recent years, partly with the change in attitudes. For example, in previous years it was a regular practice to visit all children under 5 years old with a fever; this no longer takes place as a routine, partly because of changes in social circumstances whereby more people have access to transport or their own cars.

Home visits are not necessarily a good thing. They are often made for what may be perceived by GPs as trivial conditions (Cartwright 1986). Clearly it takes time to see each patient and to travel between houses. It has been estimated that each GP spends about two hours every working day doing home visits. This is the equivalent to a whole surgery where 15 or more patients may be seen; consequently between 50 and 100 extra appointments could be made at the surgery if visits were not done during this two-hour time span. In addition, on home visits, specialised equipment may not be available — ECGs, nebulisers, glucose monitoring kits, etc. A certain amount of equipment can be carried by the GP, but clearly she or he cannot carry everything and thus a short consultation in an unsatisfactory home environment with inadequate equipment, under pressure of time, may mean that a home visit is not an appropriate way of performing modern British general practice.

Out-of-hours work Full-time general practitioners are paid for providing a continuous service to their patients. Incorporated within this are out-of-hours responsibilities, that is on-call commitments at evenings and night-times and over weekends. Arrangements for these 24 hours a day, 365 days a year commitments vary. The terms of service state that 'the doctor shall give treatment personally to the patient unless reasonable steps are taken to ensure continuity of treatment by another doctor acting as a deputy'. The average size of practice is now between three and four principals per partnership, and thus most partnerships will elect to do their own on-call rota or share a rota with a neighbouring practice.

The alternative to this is for part or all of the on-call duties to be done using a deputising service. Approval for this must be obtained from the FHSA.

There are advantages and disadvantages to each system of organising out-of-hours cover. From the patient's point of view, seeing their own doctor is a great advantage. This is someone who is known and trusted, is aware of their problems, lives locally and will get to them speedily. From the GPs' point of view, the advantage of providing the service themselves is that they know the patients and can get to them quickly. Knowing the problems may mean that a telephone call will be all that is necessary; equally it may be clear from the GP's previous knowledge that immediate assistance is required. Out-of-hours work can be perceived as a source of education and satisfaction for the GP (Iliffe & Haug 1991). Furthermore, there is a financial incentive in that a visit requested and carried out between 10 p.m. and 8 a.m. the following morning attracts a night visit fee.

The disadvantage is the unsocial nature of the work which, in addition to being stressful on top of a full day's work, is also tiring and can lead to a reduced standard of performance in the next day's surgery, with consequent medical risks for the patient and medico-legal risks for the doctor.

It may be possible to reduce these particular problems by providing a recovery period for a doctor who has been on duty, for example by cancelling morning surgeries after a night on-call for the doctor concerned. Alternatively the doctor may choose to use a deputising service. This has the advantages of reducing unsocial out-of-hours commitment, reducing levels of tiredness, and allowing better performance in the surgery and during the day. In areas where visiting is not safe — usually in inner cities — then it may be safer to use a deputising service where unaccompanied visits are not done and where there is ready access to radio and CB help.

The disadvantages are that the deputising service may cover a very wide area and so may not be practical in any other than a city environment because the length of time between the visit being requested and that visit being done may be unacceptably long, running into hours rather than minutes. In addition, there is a financial disadvantage in that a deputising service has to be paid for, and any visits done by a service between the hours of 10 p.m. and 8 a.m. attract a reduced night visit fee of one-third the standard fee. The calculation is not that straightforward as clearly this cost is allowable against tax and, in addition, there may be an increased number of visits because the deputising service is more likely to visit than the patient's own doctor.

There has been considerable debate as to the future of out-of-hours work. A recent survey found that a majority of GPs would like to opt out of the 24-hour commitment. Alternative arrangements may need to be considered. Suggestions have been made for emergency centres covering a population of 100 000 or more, staffed by groups of GPs banding together or an NHS deputising service. These proposals will need to be considered and discussed by both the profession and the Government in view of implications for care and the costs involved.

DISCUSSION POINT

Out-of-hours work

In hospital practice the bulk of the 'on-call' work is done by the junior doctors. With a few exceptions, when a doctor reaches consultant level, he or she can expect to have an undisturbed night's sleep. The only speciality consistently to operate a shift system is the Accident and Emergency system.

— Should general practitioners operate a shift system for out-of-hours work?
— What implications does this idea have for numbers of GPs in the country, size of partnerships, practice organisation and cost to the NHS?
— How would this affect the service given to patients?
— What other options could be realistically considered?

Health advice

GPs are expected to provide health advice within the consultation. This seems an eminently sensible idea but probably only a small proportion of consulting time is devoted to this. Furthermore, it is not clear that it has any significant long-term effects on patient behaviour. It is more likely that social and cultural expectations as a whole have greater influence than a visit to the doctor.

The reasons for this are open to debate. It is possible that the lack of interest shown by some doctors in primary health care and health promotion is responsible. It may be that some patients do not feel that any action they can take will influence their health and have a 'fatalistic' attitude to illness and disease (Pill & Stott 1982). Perhaps busy GPs simply do not have the time to devote to giving health advice.

For these reasons it seems likely that considerable effort and time would need to be devoted to health promotion to achieve measurable changes in patient behaviour. This seems an ideal activity for delegation, along with vaccination, to a suitably trained practice nurse. This is exactly what seems to be happening as the number of practice nurses has risen dramatically in recent years (there are now about 13 000 practice nurses in England and Wales).

Under the 1990 GP contract there was an incentive to set up organised health promotion clinics. These attracted a fee of £45 each provided they were approved by the FHSA, followed a protocol, were held on a regular basis and attracted the required minimum of patients. Additionally there was an obligation to invite all patients not seen within the previous three years and offer them a physical examination.

From March 1993 the oganisation of health promotion will change. Three-yearly checks will be abandoned. From 1st July 1992 to 31st March 1993 there is a ceiling on clinic sessions, based on the number of remunerated sessions which a practice has held from 1st March 1992 to 31st May 1992. After March 1993 payment for clinics will be scrapped — with the exception of diabetes and asthma clinics, which will be classified as chronic disease management clinics. In place of this, remuneration for health promotion will be based on the Government's white paper *Health of the Nation*, which specifies five key areas in which substantial improvement in health are to be achieved. These are:

(i) Coronary heart disease and stroke
(ii) Cancers
(iii) Mental illness
(iv) HIV/AIDS and sexual health
(v) Accidents.

Practices will be streamed into separate bands according to how far they meet local health promotion objectives. Initially the banding will apply to the first of the key areas specified in the *Health of the Nation* white paper. Later, it is likely to apply also to the other key objectives. For coronary heart disease prevention the requirements are as follows:

Band 1 — recording of height, weight, body mass index, blood pressure and smoking habits in an agreed percentage of the target group.

Band 2 — as for Band 1 but a higher proportion of the target group will have to have measurements recorded. Exercise, healthy life style and dietary advice should be given.

Band 3 — as for Bands 1 and 2 but a still higher percentage of patients will have to be covered. In addition, other key areas in the white paper should be addressed.

Each practice will apply to its FHSA for admission to the band of its choice and the level of targets will depend on the practice band, with a ceiling on the payments that can be received. The contents of clinics will be based on national objectives and local needs, the latter decided after discussion with the FHSAs.

Exactly how objectives will be met, targets agreed, and recording monitored has yet to be clearly defined. It seems likely that some innovative ideas for health promotion will be shelved and opportunistic screening again become acceptable. Whether this will result in health promotion objectives being met 'better', or more fully, remains to be seen.

Vaccinations

GPs are required to offer to patients, where appropriate, vaccination or immunisation against measles, mumps, rubella, pertussis, poliomyelitis, diphtheria and tetanus. This is another excellent area where workload can be delegated to the practice nurse.

It is also potentially financially rewarding. These vaccinations attract a fee as an item of service. In addition, if the vaccines are bought by the practice, then their cost can be reclaimed with an oncost container allowance which means that a small profit will be made on each immunisation.

(Finally, for the childhood vaccinations, there is a fee if certain target levels are reached in the specified age ranges, which are for primary immunisations to be given before the age of three, and boosters to be given before the age of six.)

It may not be easy to reach a target, however. Firstly, it is necessary to know exactly how many children are in the target age range. This may sound simple enough but in an area with a highly mobile population there may be a turnover of more than 15% annually. Newly registered patients may not have kept their immunisation details so it may be necessary to contact their previous GP. Other people may have left the area without notifying the practice, in which case contacting them may prove impossible. This may not matter in the sense that the FHSA can be notified that these people have moved ('ghosts'!) but it can make reaching targets extremely difficult. In addition, the practice lists may not correlate with those of the FHSA, further complicating the process.

Not all parents may wish their children to be vaccinated. Certain cultural and ethnic populations may have particular, especially religious, reasons for declining immunisation. Some people do not realise the importance of the procedure and others may simply be too busy to get around to having it done. Finally there is a residual feeling that vaccination may be dangerous:

this is mostly a 'hangover' effect from a number of cases of brain damage, at the time thought to result from the pertussis vaccine in the late 1960s and early 1970s.

It seems reasonable, therefore, to make attempts to inform people of the value of immunisation and to make it easily available. The practice nurse is in an ideal position to seek out children requiring vaccination, perhaps with the help of the health visitor. An up-to-date practice register, with adequate records of vaccination details and secretarial and medical support, is essential if targets are to be reached.

Clearly, if the practice nurse does all the work she should be suitably valued and commensurately paid. Sticking needles into screaming children all day long requires care, compassion and patience. Equally, this is a clinical area where things can go wrong. The nurse should be suitably trained, and insured both directly under nursing insurance and also by the practice through a medical defence society.

DISCUSSION POINT

Vaccination

It seems reasonable to make every attempt to vaccinate as many children as possible. However, what do you do if there is one family that persistently refuses to have *their* child vaccinated and this prevents the practice from reaching a target level, perhaps costing the practice thousands of pounds per year?

— What options are open to you?

— What is the ethical basis for your decision?

— In France parents are paid a fee for having their children vaccinated and in the USA it is a legal requirement for vaccinations to be completed before a child can attend school. Should the Government drop targets as part of general practice and instead adopt a system of making parents rather than doctors responsible for having their children vaccinated?

B. Additional services

GPs may also provide contraceptive services, child health surveillance services, minor surgery services and maternity medical services to any person, as well as general medical services. They can do so only if they have previously undertaken and been accepted to provide those services by the Family Health Services Authority. For each of these services the GP may claim a fee.

Traditionally, GPs have provided contraceptive and maternity medical services. Those doctors who have obtained the family planning certificate can offer fitting of intrauterine contraceptive devices and those GPs accepted as having completed satisfactory training in obstetrics are paid a higher fee for doing so by the FHSA. Similarly, only those GPs who have completed the necessary training and have been approved by the FHSA can offer child health surveillance and minor surgery services.

There are particular requirements for the provision of each of these services and problems associated with their implementation. In the case of child health surveillance the GP must be on the FHSA child health surveillance list. The patient must be under 5 years old and the GP must provide child health surveillance according to a programme agreed by the FHSA and DHA or health board.

To organise this properly, there must be enough space in the surgery. The room needs to be a suitable size, well sound-proofed, and arranged so that children can be examined in comfort, with their parents present and over a long enough period of time. There must be enough space in the waiting room for the families or even a separate reception area. The work must be planned so that it takes place regularly over the course of the year. Follow-up of children with problems has to be arranged and a system of tracing defaulters put in place.

The aim of setting minimum requirements is to improve the quality of service offered. It is reasoned that the various 'tests' will ensure that minimum standards of competence and care are achieved and there is a substantial financial incentive to undertake the necessary training and pass whatever hurdle is required in order to be awarded the requisite certificate.

This trend towards more diplomas may herald a major change in the philosophy of general practice. By creating an increasing number of examinations to be passed, this system may result in specialisation of doctors so that each doctor may become an 'expert' in a particular field. Within a practice there may be one doctor who performs minor surgery, another who does the child health surveillance and a different GP responsible for family planning.

There is no reason for the separation of doctors by specialisation to stop there. Why not have a specialist in diabetes or an expert in

---

DISCUSSION POINT

Additional services

Until a few years ago child health surveillance was done by suitably trained medical officers in conjunction with health visitors at health authority clinics. More may be performed by GPs now that payment is being offered for this service. Most GPs now provide family planning advice.

— Who should provide these services?

— Is there any future for health authority clinics?

— What will be achieved if they are closed down?

— And what may be lost?

hormone replacement therapy? This may only be a formal extension of a situation that already exists. GPs have always tended to have their own areas of expertise. These can bring a contrast to the 'routine' work and help prevent boredom and burnout. Perhaps this is the future of general practice?

C. Recalls

The 1990 GP contract requires GPs to offer and carry out various checks on the patients registered with them. These checks are for new patients and those over 75 years old. The details of the examinations for new patients are contained in the contract (Department of Health 1989). I shall briefly describe the contractual requirements then discuss the implications that follow.

a. New patients

Newly registered patients should be offered a consultation with the GP within 20 days of acceptance on to that doctor's list. In the course of that consultation the doctor will seek details from that patient as to medical history and offer to undertake a physical examination. These consultations should be offered to any new patient aged 5 years or over and must be carried out within 3 months of them joining the practice list.

b. Over-75 checks

Patients aged 75 years and over should be invited, in each period of 12 months beginning on 1st April in each year, to participate in a consultation and offered a domiciliary visit for the purpose of assessing whether personal services need to be rendered to that patient. The assessment will include sensory functions, mobility, mental condition, physical condition including continence, social environment and the use of medicines.

Recall implications

These checks have implications for resources. They require a recall system to be set up, letters to be sent, and follow-up of response arranged. This costs money and takes time.

In order to send letters to a target group it is first necessary to identify who it comprises. This means that an age-sex register, either manual or computerised, is essential. A letter then has to be devised and sent to those who are in this group, and arrangements have to be made for the checks to be carried out.

This can involve a tremendous amount of work. How are you going to manage doing all these new patient and over-75 checks?

The obvious answer is to delegate, a skill notorious in general practice by its absence. A computer can carry all the data. Staff can enter details of all consultations and arrange for letters to be sent to target groups using a mail-merge facility on a good wordprocessing package. The checks can all be carried out by a suitably qualified person, probably a practice nurse, following a protocol agreed with the partners. This is still going to cost money in employing extra staff and requires space on the premises for the work to be carried out. It does, however, prevent valuable and expensive medical time from being wasted.

> **DISCUSSION POINT**
>
> **Recalls**
>
> — GPs are paid for doing new patient checks; can you refuse to register these patients if they do not attend for this?
> — Are nurses qualified to carry out the checks?
> — What evidence is there that over-75 checks are of any medical value?
> — What is the legal situation if you refuse to carry out checks that you believe to be valueless?
> — What is the moral situation if you carry out checks that you feel are useless?

D. Records and reports

Records

A doctor is required to:

a. keep adequate records of the illnesses and treatment of his patients,
b. forward such records to the FHSA on request as soon as possible, and
c. within 14 days of being informed by the FHSA of the death of a person on his list, forward his records relating to that person to the committee.

This requirement allows for continuity of care through the records, both between different doctors in the same practice and, if a patient moves, between different doctors in different practices. At least it is supposed to!

Doctors are notorious for their appalling handwriting. Partly this is attributable to pressure of work and partly to sheer laziness. It cannot be conducive to good medical care, however, not to be able to read someone else's writing, or even, in some cases, your own! Equally, it is essential for medico-legal reasons to keep good quality records. In these days of increasing litigation — a GP can expect one or two formal complaints during his or her medical career — your defence may rest entirely upon the quality of the notes kept at the time. As complaints can be made some time after a problem situation, and as these cases can take years to come to fruition, it is sensible not to rely on memory with no contemporaneous written supportive evidence. Lack of good quality notes has made many a case indefensible.

Furthermore, it is sound advice to be careful when writing notes. From the end of 1991 patients are legally entitled to see their records *from that date*. Additionally, the Data Protection Act allows patients to look at all information about them kept on computer (a fee can be charged for providing this information).

Even if you can read the notes you may not actually have them. The system as it stands does not even allow for rapid transfer of records from one practice to another. When patients join a new practice they complete a registration form which then has to be sent to the FHSA. The previous practice is then notified by the FHSA and the records requested. If the patients have moved area the previous FHSA has to be notified first. Eventually — and this can take several months — the notes will reach the new doctor via the (new) FHSA. This system is unsatisfactory as vital information influencing diagnosis and treatment may not be available. Of course it is possible to write to or telephone the previous doctor for the contents of the records, but this is time consuming and would be expensive to do for all new patients.

DISCUSSION POINT

Records

Where does the future lie?

Perhaps all records could be kept on computer? Then data could be transmitted countrywide via modems, on networks of compatible computers. The data would be up-to-date, legible, easily stored and readily retrieved. Or could patients keep all their own records, either as notes or on computer-compatible 'smart' cards?

— What assumptions do these suggestions make?

— What problems, e.g. of ethics, cost, privacy, may arise?

— What other options could be considered?

Prescribing and dispensing

The requirements of the 1990 GP Contract are explicit. It states that 'A doctor shall order any drugs which are needed for the treatment of any patient to whom he is providing treatment under the terms of services, by issuing to that patient a prescription form'. Clearly this is a fundamental part of being a doctor. It is also vital to understand that, as in the rest of the job, it is *the doctor's* responsibility. Thus you, *the doctor*, must sign the prescription yourself. If someone else, e.g. a receptionist, writes a prescription and you sign it, and if something goes terribly wrong, like a mistake in dosage, then it is *the doctor* who will be held to account.

As further duties are devolved to nurse practitioners this situation may change. In the future there may be changes which allow nurses to prescribe for 'minor' ailments, or for district nurses to prescribe dressings and so forth.

Practice leaflet

It is a requirement of the 1990 GP Contract that a practice leaflet is produced and made available to the patients. This document should include considerable information about the practice including personal and professional details of the doctor, practice information including the times available for consultation, use of the appointments system and methods of obtaining home visits, out-of-hours arrangements, information regarding clinics and availability of maternity medical services, etc. (Department of Health 1989).

At present most people choose their doctor by such criteria as location (Salisbury 1989). Clearly, as a patient, it is important to find a doctor who you can trust *and* who provides the services you need. A well-prepared practice leaflet should enable an informed choice to be made. In addition, it may also help long-standing patients of the practice to find out about services that can be provided within the practice. It does, however, raise a number of interesting points.

What can or cannot be included? It is illegal at present for doctors to say that they are the best GPs in the country and that the doctors down the road should never have been allowed to set up in practice. Is it allowable to say that you provide a first-class quality service? If so, how are you going to measure this?

Where can you put your practice leaflet? Certainly it can be left on the practice premises. Is it permissible though to leave it in the local library, in the county council clinic, or with the estate agent in the high street?

Producing a publication of any sort uses resources, principally time and money. Consequently, it seems logical to try and reduce those costs by obtaining some form of sponsorship, for example, from local businesses. Is it morally acceptable to obtain this funding from a drug company or allow advertising by a local chemist?

Thus the production of a practice leaflet can bring its own problems. Nevertheless, it also brings an opportunity to display to the world the type of service that *you* wish to provide, and can offer an intriguing insight into the practice and the people who work in it.

Annual reports

A report must be provided annually to the FHSA by the doctor, relating to the provision by him or her of personal medical services. This will contain information on the following:

1. staff numbers and duties
2. details of practice premises
3. referral of patients to specialists
4. the doctor's other commitments as medical practitioner
5. arrangements for patients' comments on the provision of general medical services
6. use of formularies and repeat prescriptions.

A practice report requires the collection of information by the practice and is a statutory obligation of the contract. This is a chance to look at what you are doing, to obtain an overview of what is going on and, from this, to reflect on how things can be done better, or changed. It is a management tool for yourself and the practice, and tells you a lot about the practice. It can only be of use, however, if the information collected is accurate. This requires disease registers, an accurate count of referrals and procedures done. In addition, it requires use of time and resources to compile, time that could be spent otherwise, for example in seeing patients.

Education

The 1990 contract stipulates that, for a full-time general practitioner, at least 26 hours consulting time is made available over at least 5 days a week, for a minimum of 42 weeks a year. This stipulation was made in order to prevent the situation of GPs nominally being full time but actually available to patients on a limited basis. (A common perception is that of GPs playing golf for most of the week!)

This requirement would make it very difficult for GPs to continue pursuing other interests which take up one day a week or more. In particular, much academic work and postgraduate education in general practice is conducted on a part-time basis. The 1990 GP Contract therefore has a section which states that under exceptional circumstances 'the FHSA may agree that a doctor may be available for only 4 days a week'. The day off may be taken for health-related activities including 'the organisation of the medical profession or the training of its members', which means that people such as vocational Training Course Organisers have been able to continue their educational role.

Although there have been some obstacles placed in the way of GPs *providing* continuing education, by contrast there has been a revolution in the methods by which GPs *obtain* it. The Postgraduate Education

Allowance (PGEA) is paid to GPs who have attended the requisite number of approved educational sessions over the preceding year. Basically, the full amount is paid for attendance at 10 sessions — for practical purposes this works out as 10 half days — in the areas of health promotion, disease management and service management. As the sum is more than £2000 there has been a rush from GPs to attend courses of all types. The regulations have some flexibility too, so that it is possible to attend lunchtime meetings (usually approved for $\frac{1}{3}$ session) over a 12-month period and still be eligible for the full PGEA.

This system is not immune from criticism however. 'Signing up' at a course does not guarantee learning anything at all. Attendance to qualify for money does not necessarily equate with motivation to learn. The increase in number of courses may offer a wider choice of subject matter but may mean a reduction in quality of material. Although all courses still have to be approved by the Regional Advisor (or Postgraduate Dean in Wales) there may also be a conflict of interest. Regional Advisors are not only responsible for ensuring that GPs have access to courses but they also may be responsible for providing them. A case can be made for separating the two roles.

A final point should be made about 'incentives'. Although the PGEA is money available for attending educational activities, this is not 'new' money. The finance has come from other parts of the GP's budget. Thus, obtaining this allowance merely allows a GP to maintain his or her own income. Failure to qualify for the PGEA will result in a *reduction* in income. In other words, GPs are penalised for not going

---

DISCUSSION POINT

Postgraduate education allowance (PGEA)

In order to claim this GPs must have completed 5 days of accredited postgraduate education over the preceding year. It is assumed that attending for educational activities on a regular basis enables GPs to maintain their knowledge and skill levels.

— What does this system intend and what is actually happening?

— Does attendance equate with learning?

— How do GPs learn?

— What evidence is available that GPs have become 'better informed' and more 'up-to-date' since 1990?

— What other options for continuing postgraduate medical education for GPs could be considered.

— Would (re)accreditation be a more satisfactory method of ensuring that GPs keep up-to-date?

on courses. Surely it would be better to *reward* those GPs who pursue self-directed adult learning?

II. ORGANISATION FOR SERVICE PROVISION

Premises

Under the provision of the 1990 GP Contract GPs must allow inspection of their premises by a member or officer of the FHSA or local medical committee or both. This is intended to ensure that these premises are designed and maintained to good standards, and patients can expect to be seen in privacy and reasonable comfort.

Until the early 1960s, the majority of general practitioners consulted from their own homes. With the Doctors' Charter of 1965, there was then an incentive for GPs to band together with the advent of the group practice allowance. Furthermore, partial remuneration of staff costs meant that it was now possible to employ more people to undertake administrative and secretarial duties. Consequently, space had to be increased to provide for this. Thus there was a shift towards more centralised premises and the use of converted or purpose-built premises. The majority of general practice now takes place from such buildings. The major decisions for the practice therefore will involve the structure of the premises and whether these should be owned or rented.

Clearly the size of the premises needs to allow for consulting, examination, a waiting area and room to keep records and equipment. There also needs to be a room for employed staff to work. Thus for a practice of three GPs, it may be necessary to have three consulting rooms, each perhaps with its own examination area or examination room, a treatment room for a practice nurse if employed, a waiting room, a reception area, an area for storage of records, perhaps a filing room and a room for the secretaries and possibly a practice manager, in addition to any other storage rooms and toilets.

Location

The practice needs to be located where the majority of patients have easy access. This may not be so important if the practice is in an area where there is a high car-owner population, but certainly requires careful consideration where this is not the case; access by public transport then becomes extremely important. It has been shown that the location of the general practice in relation to the patient's home is the most important factor in choosing a GP (Salisbury 1989). With the increasing competition envisaged by the new GP contract of 1990, this may become less important. With perhaps 200 consultations or more occurring every day, room for car parking is essential. Staff, doctors and patients visiting to pick up repeat prescriptions, make appointments and make enquiries, etc., also need to be considered.

Structure

Converted premises have the disadvantage of a design not suited to the purpose. They may be cramped throughout, or have some rooms which are very large and others which are too small. There may be inadequate space for consulting, leading to partners sharing rooms and potential chaos. Despite the structure of the building not necessarily suiting its function, the atmosphere may well be more conducive to good general practice (as discussed in Ch. 4).

In an ideal world it might be envisaged that a purpose-built surgery with specifically designed consulting and examination rooms would be extremely desirable. Certainly this was felt to be the case in the 1960s and early 1970s when a large number of health centres were built and funds were readily available. However, a health centre may also have disadvantages. If it is local authority owned, they may have no incentive to maintain the buildings, to improve the structure or even to redecorate. It may be necessary to create a real fuss before anything is done. If two practices are occupying the same health centre, they may have different priorities, both of staff and organisation. One practice may not care what is done: all the responsibilities and duties of maintenance may then devolve almost by default to the other practice. There may be differences of opinion as to the necessity for capital expenditure or disputes over the cost of maintenance such that, on a trivial level, there may be major disputes simply over getting a building redecorated.

A practice may decide that it is worth building its own premises. This is a major undertaking requiring considerable time, energy and money. As with any major construction project, it requires planning permission, architects, solicitors, as well as the actual construction work. It is also financially a major proposition with costs exceeding one million pounds in some cases.

Reimbursement is available under the cost-rent regulation. This scheme exists basically to enable general practitioners to build new premises without being financially crippled. Within limits, the FHSA will pay the interest on the loan whilst the general practice bears the costs of the capital repayments. Above these limits the GPs pay the capital costs *and* the interest on this.

The scheme does not apply in the same way to the conversion of premises. (Conversions attract about 60% funding of the interest payments whereas building new premises attracts 100% providing the special regulations in the Red Book are adhered to.) This scheme is 'the art of the possible'. Compromises need to be made on location, building materials, size of rooms and so forth. For a new building to be completed requires the goodwill of the FHSA and the district valuer. The whole process may take years to complete, put enormous strain on the partners and affect the way the partnership functions. The new financial burden entails responsibilities that must be enshrined in the partnership agreement. Partners may be found muttering in corners years later discussing the cost and problems of toilet fittings.

Owner-occupied versus rented accommodation

Rented premises have the advantage that there is no capital risk attached to them. It means that a new incoming partner does not have to find what may be a large sum of money in order to pay the outgoing partner for his/her share in the practice premises. It also means that should a decision be made to leave the premises, they do not have to be sold with the problems and cost that this entails. Responsibility for the maintenance of the building will then fall to the owner of that building. However, there may be problems with disposal of an unexpired lease.

Checklist for trainees

In your practice:

- Is the location easy to get to for patients?
- Is it on a bus or train route?
- Is there space for car parking?
- Are the premises purpose-built or converted?
- How much space is available?
- Is there a room for a nurse?
- Is there a separate room for the trainee?
- Is there space for equipment and notes?
- Are the premises well maintained?

DISCUSSION POINT

Premises

Financing new premises through the cost-rent scheme is thought to be an excellent way to improve the quality of surgery accommodation. Is there any evidence that this is the case? Funds are limited and likely to become more so. There are complicated regulations governing size of rooms, etc., which constrain development.

— Should the cost-rent scheme be abolished?

— What alternatives to financing the building of new premises are available?

— Should the Government make direct grants to GPs towards the cost of improving premises?

— What are the possible complications of adopting this option?

Owned premises have almost the flip-side of this as their advantages. Although in the early years paying for the premises may prove costly, there may be capital appreciation over a period of time. Most of the value of this is likely to be in the land and not in the building itself. This may be quite substantial and amount to a nest-egg for the retiring GP. Additionally, it means that the partners can make and decide on alterations to the premises between themselves, without having to negotiate through a third party.

For both renting and owning premises, there is reimbursement of the cost. The assessment is done by the District Valuer, who is employed by the FHSA. In the case of renting, this is direct reimbursement of the cost of the rent. In the case of owning, it is either a notional rent based upon the likely cost of renting comparable premises or the interest on the actual cost incurred in building new premises. There may be problems in reaching agreement over reimbursement, for example in inner cities where commercial rates distort valuations, in which case the practice is entitled to appeal.

Staff

Could you manage without your receptionist? Could you do the job as well as he or she does? Why are most receptionists women? (This is supposed to be an age of equality!) Could you face dealing with irate members of the public who complain that they can't see their doctor for days and days? Who would take this sort of poorly paid job and tolerate the difficulties that it may bring with it?

There must be advantages to the job or GPs wouldn't be able to get any staff at all! So why do people work as receptionists, what are they expected to do? Are they disposable lackeys or indispensable members of a team? Do they act to protect the doctor from 'difficult' patients or enable worried and ill people to get access to a medical service?

From the general practitioner's viewpoint, staff are needed to implement both the spirit and the letter of the 1990 contract, to help provide a service to the patients in organising administration, to help provide good quality medical care with easy access for the patients to doctors, nurses and staff, and to enable the GPs to fulfil their business role, i.e. to earn a living. It is clear that different staff are needed for these different tasks although there may be considerable overlap. A brief list of staff required may be as follows:

- Receptionist
- Telephonist
- Filing clerk
- Secretary
- Computer operator
- Practice nurses
- Practice manager.

This is not a comprehensive list of staff. The numbers employed by different practices vary or may vary in the same practice over a period of time, depending on finances, availability of suitably qualified staff, changing health needs and changing contractual requirements. Nor is the role of different staff members necessarily mutually exclusive, for example, receptionists may often share some switchboard duties or help with the filing, and the practice nurses may need to be computer-literate if there is a computer in the practice, to enter diagnosis, items of service, complete forms, etc. Most of the tasks that they perform could be performed by the doctors, but clearly it is not an appropriate use of expensive medical time to be continually filing and drawing notes. Thus, in many ways, the jobs that are performed may be looked upon as a delegation of function by the employing GPs in order to provide an effective and efficient medical service and to run a properly organised business.

The previous contract stated that up to two full-time members of staff (or whole-time equivalents) might be employed and reimbursed for each full-time partner in general practice. The partnership would be reimbursed up to a maximum of 70% of the staff salary according to agreed scales, which are generally Whitley Council scales, by the Family Health Services Authority. This was a maximum number in terms of reimbursement. Of course, there was nothing to prevent the practice employing more than this number of staff, although they would not have received any of the cost of these additional people back from the FHSA. Furthermore, there was nothing to stop a practice paying more than the Whitley Council scales although this additional cost again would not be reimbursed. Despite these incentives GPs currently employ just over one whole-time equivalent staff member for each full-time practitioner, despite the marginal cost on this basis of employing more people, especially if tax relief is taken into account. This surely must be a short-sighted policy leading to increased pressure on all those working in the practice. It makes it difficult to provide the best possible service and additionally reduces job satisfaction for all concerned.

There are now no such rules; GPs negotiate directly with the FHSA and may be able to obtain full reimbursement for staff employed. However, it is unlikely that the FHSA would agree to increase funding for existing staff. It is more probable that they would agree to extra funding for new staff employed on a specific basis, especially if they could be shown to be improving the quality of care to the patients or implementing particular agreed policies such as entering data onto computer in order to establish disease registers, etc. Thus there are now huge opportunities to improve services offered to patients by suitable employment of staff. Reimbursement will be between 0% and 100% and is dependent on being able to show that all staff employed are necessary for their particular functions.

Most staff are not full-time, nor do they work in practice solely for the money, because the pay is not very good compared to commercial rates of pay which may be obtained for similar types of office work. Generally it appears that the general practice environment provides a feeling of helping other people, a social contact and also perhaps a little prestige.

There are arguments both for and against having full-time staff. Full-timers get to know their way around the work very well and perhaps acquire expertise, for example in dealing with difficult situations at the reception desk or on the telephone. They provide continuity of service and of care both for the patients and other staff as well as the doctors. However, when they are away for whatever reason, whether sickness or holiday, then this provides more of a gap that has to be covered, either by taking on additional temporary staff or increasing the workload of other staff in the practice. The danger is then that some other necessary jobs get postponed or simply are not done. There is also differing legal status in this country between full-time and part-time staff, in that staff working more than 16 hours a week are entitled to redundancy payments and are covered by the terms of employment legislation so that, for example, set procedures have to be followed if firing a full-time member staff is contemplated. In these circumstances it is necessary to issue at least one verbal warning and one written warning prior to termination of employment. Thus it is wise to set down a contract which provides safeguards for both parties, the employer and the employee, in the event of a dispute or question over terms of employment arising. It provides a much more secure background against which people can carry out their jobs. It is also sensible to provide a written job description (see Appendix I) at the time of employing staff so that it is quite clear what job he or she is expected to do, and so that there is reduced risk of disputes occurring over duties to be done once the person has actually started.

Training, in some form, should be provided for the staff. In many ways general practice is unique, with its contacts with people requiring health advice who are often very anxious and distressed. Often there is no formal training whatsoever of staff on entering the practice and as such they are thrown in at the deep end, causing problems both for the patients and for the new and established members of staff. It behoves GPs to remember that they are legally responsible for the people they employ. If a member of staff makes an error, for example by giving inappropriate advice to a patient who subsequently becomes ill, or not making necessary arrangements for people to be seen by the doctors, then a complaint may ensue. This can result in a GP being called to a Service Committee hearing. These cases may only represent a small number of the total complaints about general practitioners but they are nevertheless a very important area which should not be neglected.

Studies of receptionists' views about training have shown that they feel themselves to be poorly trained and to be taken for granted (Copeman & Van Swanenburg 1988). Receptionists themselves view their role as helping the patient, providing access of the patient to the doctor. There is no doubt that some receptionists view their principal role as protecting the GP from 'difficult patients' and, if they are viewed by the patients as stopping access to the doctors, then understandably they will be resented and viewed as an interference with medical care and looked upon as 'dragons behind the desk' (Arber & Sawyer 1985). They have a difficult job to do; they look to, and need support from, the doctors who are also their employers. It therefore seems common sense to look after your staff.

The advent of a practice administrator or practice manager has further aided GPs in delegation of responsibilities. A competent practice manager will be able to relieve GPs of much of the burden of administrative duties by looking after, for example, staff salaries, maintenance of buildings, ordering of drugs and equipment, and so forth. Furthermore, a practice manager may be able to help with development of practice activities, whether this is expansion as a business or of premises, introduction of new equipment, employing new staff, or expanding the range of medical services offered. For the practice manager to do this, though, he or she must necessarily have access to a lot of information on how the practice is run, the state of the finances, the plans of the partners, and so on. The position may consequently be a difficult one. Partners may be reluctant to provide what is regarded as sensitive information about future plans for practice development or partners' income, or be reluctant to involve the practice manager when there is a partnership dispute. Without trust and mutual understanding, it will be almost impossible for the practice manager to perform the job. Furthermore, if the practice manager has responsibility for hiring and firing staff, then he or she may also come into contact with the other employees in the practice and be seen as a blunt tool of 'the management'. In these circumstances it is vital that he or she has the support and confidence of the partners; if decisions taken are then impeded or reversed by the partners, the practice manager's position will be severely undermined.

DISCUSSION POINT

Practice manager

A practice manager may make important decisions influencing the running of the practice, introducing policies which increase practice revenue, and acting in a proactive manner using his or her own initiative. In this situation the practice manager is assuming many of the responsibilities which would previously have been shared by the partners.

— Should the practice manager be made a full profit-sharing partner?

— What are the arguments for and against this?

— Does it make sense to have a practice manager at all? Would it make more sense to delegate all these responsibilities to one of the partners in return for a reduction in clinical commitments — an executive partner?

Although the practice manager may be able to settle a lot of the problems and disputes which may arise from time to time, it is important that the staff feel they can have access to the partners to reflect back on changes that may have occurred in the practice, the way the practice is running, to be able to provide ideas and suggestions and to air grievances, if appropriate. It would seem sensible, then, for the partners to keep in touch with the feelings and views of their staff, either on an individual formal or informal basis, or by regular practice meetings. The relationship between staff and doctors is an important one, and the happiness or otherwise of the practice is likely to be reflected in the approach to patients and their needs.

The primary health care team

The list of people closely involved with GPs in their care for a practice population is clearly not confined just to staff employed by the practice. The concept of the primary health care team came about in the early 1960s and has been extended and refined since then through the Cumberlege Report (Department of Health and Social Security 1986) and now with the 1990 GP Contract (Department of Health 1989). The definition may be rather imprecise, but other professionals and health care individuals include social workers, community psychiatric nurses, district nurses, health visitors, etc. A wider definition might include the home care team, physiotherapists, occupational therapists and so forth.

Ideally the primary health care team should function in an efficient and coordinated manner, such that actions of individuals or organisations are not duplicated and that services provided are complementary and appropriate to the needs of an individual or community. For example, an elderly person at home, immobile with leg ulcers, senile dementia and heart failure, might require the services of the GP for medical needs, the community psychiatric nurse for psychiatric problems, the health visitor for the elderly or social worker to organise social needs or provision of extra funds, the district nurses to care for the leg ulcers, the occupational therapist to provide hand rails for the bath and toilet, and the domiciliary physiotherapist to maintain mobility. This sort of activity requires close coordination and regular communication between the members of the primary health care team. This could be by telephone but is usually better face to face; this is then dependent on regular meetings being arranged.

Sometimes this sort of teamwork seems to work well, sometimes it does not. For regular meetings of this number of people to take place there has to be a suitable venue, time has to be set aside, probably an agenda organised and a chairperson appointed. There has to be a good relationship and a free exchange of ideas and information between the various individuals of the team, and feedback on the end-results. If the motivation of any of these individuals is not high, then the team is not likely to function well. Furthermore, it may be difficult to arrange mutually convenient times. Time taken for these meetings may have to come out of time used for other activities such as direct contact with patients. A suitable venue may be impossible to find.

Additionally, there may be some conflict between the various carers concerned, such that one individual sees his/her role as being usurped by another from a different part of the health care team. Under these circumstances fragmentation and disintegration of the primary health care team may occur, leading to recriminations and poor use of resources. Thus, what is ideal may not be attainable and the best that can be hoped for is a realistic, practical compromise, with individual approaches being used to individual problems. The trainee should come into contact with all the members of the primary health care team, as well all the staff, at various stages of the year, and should have a first-hand opportunity to discover the attributes and limitations of the people involved and their relationships with each other. In a happy atmosphere there is likely to be more exchange of information and ideas with all the people involved, and this is likely to shape both the way the trainee thinks about staff and health care organisation, and the way she or he behaves with respect to the organisation in the future. If no-one speaks to the trainee or helps him or her with problems this could make for a very difficult year, even with a good relationship with the trainer and the other doctors in the practice, whereas a happy, communicative, mutually interactive atmosphere is likely to lead to a happy trainee year.

The trainee should also not forget the effect that she or he may have on the practice and staff — someone willing to help out with the difficult problems a particular patient may have, pick up extra visits, take the overflow telephone calls, or be contributing both to the efficient running of the practice and probably to its morale as well.

Checklist for trainees

In your practice:
- How many staff are employed full or part time, and what are their skills?
- Is there a compact primary health care team?
- What is the relationship with district nurses, health visitors, etc?
- Are there regular staff meetings?
- Are there regular primary health care team meetings?
- Is there an opportunity to study the role of staff and primary health care team?
- What effect do the staff have on the trainee and vice versa?
- What is the communication and atmosphere like?

If staff are to be delegated responsibilities they must have access to medical information. This is an essential part of them being regarded as part of the team and it is essential that staff and doctors can trust each other. Therefore, they will have access to what may be regarded as sensitive information about individuals. In particular, this may include sexually transmitted diseases, including syphilis and AIDS, or potentially embarrassing situations for the patient such as terminations of unwanted pregnancies and so forth. This issue is essentially an ethical one involving confidentiality. Patients must be able to trust their doctor and, by extension, staff holding such information, not to divulge this sort of knowledge to outside individuals or agencies. There may be situations where the doctors feel that it is inappropriate for the staff to be informed of particular situations, for example, a patient with AIDS, and for most of the practice staff this may be satisfactory in that their likelihood of being exposed to an infection from such an individual is remote. However, the doctors owe a duty also to their staff; clearly the practice nurse taking blood or a district nurse involved in incontinence care is in a different situation to a receptionist making an appointment at the desk. It is a tricky ethical dilemma as to how much information can be given to the staff; it is therefore important, from the moment of appointment, that the staff understand their obligation of confidentiality to the patients. A breach of confidentiality by a doctor is a serious matter, having implications for the confidence of patients in their future medical care and being difficult to defend should a complaint be brought. By extension, this applies also to the staff employed by a practice and may be considered grounds for dismissal.

DISCUSSION POINT

Confidentiality

It is common practice to delegate responsibility to the receptionists for giving results of laboratory tests to the patients. Usually the doctors will have seen the results first and marked a response, e.g. 'normal' or 'to make appointment'. The receptionist would then tell the patient this when they telephone or come to the surgery for the result. There may be cases where this is clearly not appropriate, for example, the result of an HIV test. In other situations, such as the results of a pregnancy test, the risk to confidentiality may not be so clear cut. Perhaps though, the whole question of delegating this responsibility to members of staff needs to be examined.
— How do you know who is ringing up for a result?
— Do your staff live locally and perhaps know the person concerned or their parents?
— Perhaps *all* laboratory results should be given by the doctor directly to the patient. If so, what implications does this have for the doctor's time and its potential effect on other patients?

Morale

Good staff morale in the practice is likely to help improve service to the patients, enthusiasm towards attaining targets, etc. A review of individual and overall performance should allow areas of competence and excellence to be recognised and areas of weakness to be discussed. If mistakes are continually picked upon, and competence and achievement pass unrecognised, morale is likely to be low and staff turnover high. Recognition may be verbal or written in terms of praise: with the new targets in practice it may be relevant to consider bonuses for performance as both a reward and an incentive, in addition to the traditional party or Christmas gifts.

Equipment

Every doctor will have a view on what constitutes *essential* equipment. There is an enormous number of items that it is possible to use in general practice, and with the ever increasing changes in modern medicine this is increasing all the time. For a patient with severe asthma a nebuliser may be lifesaving. An electrocardiograph may be a vital piece of equipment in making a diagnosis in someone with chest pain, and a defibrillator will be needed for a patient in ventricular fibrillation. However, most time in general practice is spent dealing with less potentially catastrophic situations. The most essential equipment for a good GP is his or her eyes and ears and the ability to elicit and then interpret information from the patient.

There are times when additional equipment is useful. This can be divided into those items commonly used, and those which may be important less often (Table 3.2).

This list is not comprehensive; trainees are advised to look at the equipment available in the practices to which they are attached and decide for themselves what equipment they feel is essential or which they would like to have. Furthermore, some doctors would regard items such as a nebuliser as *essential* equipment, and place other items further down the list.

Table 3.2 List of equipment

Commonly used
Stethoscope
Auriscope
Ophthalmoscope
Tongue depressors
Peak flow meter
Vaginal specula
Sphygmomanometer

Less commonly used
Electrocardiograph
Nebuliser
Suturing equipment
Defibrillator

Nevertheless, it is interesting to note that most of the items used on a regular basis are for *diagnostic* purposes, whereas *treatment* equipment falls into the less often used category. This division neatly highlights the priority for any doctor, and especially for GPs, to *diagnose* first and only then, if appropriate, to offer treatment.

It will be noted that no mention has been made so far of the role, if any, of the computer. This piece of equipment, which is a relatively modern addition to the tools available to GPs, has caused considerable discussion as to its value and role in general practice. It is, therefore, suitable as an example of how decisions can be reached about the purchase and use of equipment in General Practice.

The computer

In common with all other items of equipment, it is important to ask why a computer should be required by a practice. After all, general practice has survived quite happily until now without needing such 'high tech' pieces of apparatus.

Or has it? Is this an unwarranted assumption? Is this relevant anyway? In modern general practice it is more logical to ask whether a computer is needed *now*. Why is it required? What tasks can it perform better than or in addition to existing systems? What disadvantages does it have? How much will it cost? Which one should be bought?

A computer acts as a store of information which allows ready access to and retrieval of information. It will sort data and, properly programmed, enables information to be analysed and reports to be rapidly produced.

This speed of action is probably the greatest asset of the computer. There are also drawbacks. A computer is only as good as the data entered on it, or the software provided. It requires staff to use it, so must be easy to operate, i.e. 'user friendly'. Both the computers and terminals ('hardware')

Table 3.3 The computer as equipment

Benefits	Disadvantages
List correlation	Use of space
Achieving targets	Garbage in?
Producing recall letters	Extra staff
Production of reports	Doctor-patient relationship?
Disease registers	New technology — ?scares
Acute/repeat scripts	Costs
Staff salaries	Breakdowns — reliability?

and extra staff have to be accommodated somewhere in the practice. If it is used by doctors during the consultation it increases consultation time and *may* interfere with the 'doctor-patient relationship' (although there is little evidence that it does any harm and may actually be helpful on occasion).

Thus complex decisions on the relative benefits of the computer — as with any item of equipment — have to be made (as in Table 3.3).

Using a computer in the practice also raises other ethical issues. In common with all use of information involving the public, preservation of confidentiality is a legal as well as an ethical duty. Thus all patients are entitled to a copy of the computerised records kept about them (for which a charge can be made). These rights are enshrined in the Data Protection Act which obliges GPs who store patients' records to register this use.

It is essential to have both manual and computer 'backups' in case of fire or other catastrophe, and sufficient insurance. It is also vital to have adequate support from 'experts' who can sort out problems with programmes and software. If a practice is highly dependent upon a computer and it 'goes wrong', then the whole organisation can fall into chaos. This is not a hypothetical situation: hard disk 'crashes' do occur and GPs are not immune from sabotage by computer viruses such as 'Friday 13th' or 'Michelangelo'!

Despite all the potential problems, computers may be seen as the only satisfactory way of dealing with the increasing administrative workload. If a decision is made to buy this highly specialised piece of equipment, then there is a large choice available. This decision is likely to depend on individual circumstances; as with any major purchase it is important to choose what is right for *you*. The major constraint on any purchase is likely to be cost. Direct payment for computer costs is available on a sliding scale according to list size. The payments differ according to whether the system is purchased or leased and payments are also available for maintenance and staff costs. It is cash limited.

The need for equipment of any sort is likely to change over a period of time. General practice is not a fossilised, static subject and will evolve as a

---

Checklist for trainees

Choosing a computer system:
- Take advice.
- What 'size' (speed, disk space, etc.) is needed?
- What is the cost?
- Is it reliable?
- What 'software' support is available?
- Can the system be upgraded?

reflection of a changing society. Instruments regarded as essential a hundred years ago are now museum pieces or collectors' items. Thus it is possible to envisage huge changes taking place in the equipment needed to perform competently as a GP. 'Touchscreen' computers are already available, albeit at a high price. In the future all doctors may talk directly to personalised voice-sensitive computers which will then transcribe records, print prescriptions, etc. It may no longer be necessary to keep any written records, saving time, space, and money. Who knows? It is not possible to look into the future but sometimes a good guess can be made. A wise choice of equipment, which is then used sensibly, will enable GPs to practise competent and caring medicine.

III. MONITORING AND FINANCE

This chapter has run through the contractual requirements of GPs and some of the implications of these. Clearly each GP has to fulfil the terms of the contract, whatever he or she may think about them. GPs do not act in isolation however. They have to be paid and the standard of service provided should be monitored. This is done by the FHSA.

Each GP has a contract with the FHSA (Family Health Services Authority) to provide a service for the patients on his or her list. In return for this, he or she receives remuneration. Consequently the FHSA has a pivotal role in financing and monitoring the provision of care to the population, and in ensuring that GPs comply with the requirements of the 1990 contract. It is important therefore to understand how FHSAs function.

Family Health Services Authority (FHSA)

What is the role of the FHSA? It is generally thought of as that part of the National Health Service responsible for the services provided to patients by family doctors, dentists, pharmacists and opticians. This implies that it is our (GPs') employer. This is a contradiction in terms— how is it possible for GPs to be independent contractors and yet be employed by and responsible to the FHSA? It also raises questions about the relationship between GPs and the FHSA. Are FHSAs 'facilitators', enabling an improvement in the level of services to be provided, or do they act as an enforcement agency for the Government to make sure that GPs carry out the role that has been set out for them? In the sense that every GP has signed a contract with the FHSA to provide medical services to a population then it can be looked upon as an enabler. However, the new contract was imposed on general practitioners against the wishes of most of them (and a large part of the population as a whole) and the FHSA can then be seen as an agency working for the state. Are FHSAs then political pawns, or modern innovators? How are they organised and what are their roles?

There are 98 FHSAs in England and Wales. They are responsible to (and funded by) Regional Health Authorities, and thence to the Department of Health and the Secretary of State for Health. Generally, an FHSA will have working links with the District Health Authority, Community Health Council, District Councils, County Council and Social Services, as well as a number of voluntary organisations.

The authority established by the Secretary of State for Health under the NHS Community Care Act 1990 to replace the FPC comprises a chairman appointed by the Secretary of State, and members supported by a number of staff. The members come from a variety of backgrounds: for example, Surrey FHSA comprises an FHSA chief executive (executive director), one general medical practitioner, one general dental practitioner, one nurse, one pharmacist (non-executive directors), and five lay people. This is a time of rapid change and no two FHSAs are organised in exactly the same way.

In addition to being responsible for the management of family health services in that area, the FHSA also has to ensure the adequate provision of services to assess continuing health needs in the community, and to fund the provision and development of primary health care services. It takes into account consumer opinion although it is not clear how it does this, nor is it certain that producing patient satisfaction always means that good medical care is being provided. There is considerable debate as to what actually constitutes a 'good GP' (Arber 1987, Heath 1987). Ease of access to GPs and the attitudes of the receptionists may be an important indicator of quality of care (Cartwright 1986).

The FHSA also undertakes to provide other services including a health promotion strategy, running recall programmes for cervical cancer, breast cancer, screening programmes, etc., and (important to GPs!) is responsible for remunerating the contractors for the services they provide under the terms of their contracts with the NHS.

The number of staff supporting the FHSA may be more than 100, depending on the size of the area concerned. Funds managed may run into millions. Consequently the FHSA itself may be a large organisation with its own problems of efficiency, staff management and resource allocation. Staff may become ill or not perform well, computers may break down, and all of this is likely to impinge on the relationship of the FHSA with the GPs in the area.

As the majority of the GP's income will come from the FHSA for the services that the GP provides, it is important to maintain good communication and a good working relationship. On this basis, discrepancies between lists held by GPs and FHSAs may be reconciled, and differences over target figures be adjusted and agreed upon to mutual advantage, enabling payments to GPs to be made and received on time, records to be updated and transferred to and from GP and FHSA speedily, and problems identified and resolved. These processes are on-going and vital to the organisation of general practice, its remuneration and provision of good medical care.

If the chairman is appointed by the Secretary of State, then it seems impossible to view the FHSA as a politically independent organisation; might an FHSA try to ensure that GPs carry out the wishes of the Government of the day? On this basis GPs may end up doing things that are politically expedient or popular rather than for the 'good' of the patients. Furthermore, if funds are limited and staff employed on performance-related contracts where the criteria of success include keeping down costs, then there may be difficulties for GPs in expanding services or obtaining reimbursements to which they may feel entitled. Consequently there is a real risk of conflict between GPs and FHSAs. Even if the problems described are apparent rather than real, it is the perception of injustice that will affect the attitudes of the two parties. GPs may be perceived as recalcitrant or lazy, whilst FHSAs may be thought to be withholding funds or information. The GPs may feel that if they do not 'behave' in an approved way then this will be directly reflected in their earnings. Thus the organisation as presently defined offers both the opportunities and benefits of close cooperation and the risks and hazards of potential conflict.

DISCUSSION POINT

The Family Health Services Authority

- If GPs are no longer seen as independent contractors, will they benefit from direct negotiation with provider services such as hospitals?
- If this comes about, is there a need for the FHSAs to have a role in funding?
- How would you as trainee want to see the structure for service provision altered?
- Is there any role for the FHSAs in the future
- Could they be disbanded as yet another layer of bureaucracy?

The FHSA is not the only agency with which GPs must deal. Doctors refer patients to hospitals for advice and treatment and they in turn must obtain funding from District Health Authorities. Figure 3.2 shows in simplified form the links between FHSAs, hospitals and GPs.

This is a very simple way of viewing the organisation of service provision. With the advent of fundholding general practices and Trust Hospitals responsible for their own budgets, there has been a fundamental shift in the way that finance is obtained and spending monitored. A significant number of hospitals now have trust status and an increasing number of practices are now fundholding. The proportion of the NHS that is financed in this new way is likely to increase substantially over the next few years. This can be looked upon as a *purchaser-provider split* (Hill 1991) (Fig. 3.3).

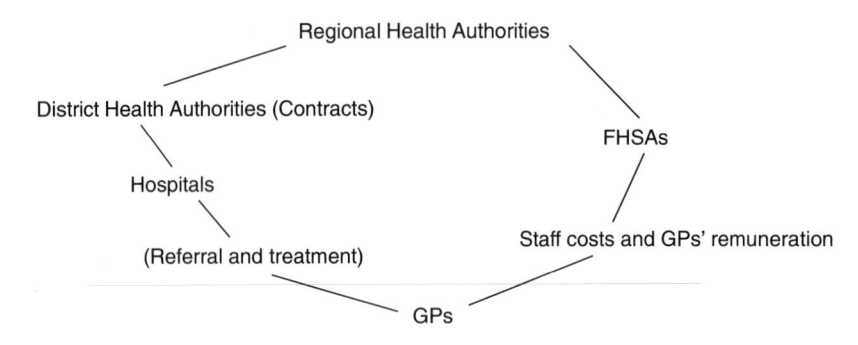

Fig. 3.2 Links between FHSAs, hospitals and GPs.

This division is an attempt to remove the conflict for health authorities in providing finance for health care as well as its delivery to the population within its geographical boundaries. Under these arrangements the health authority acts to purchase health care services for its population from providers (Fig. 3.4).

Purchasing is achieved by means of contracts. Three types of contract exist:

1. Block
2. Cost and volume
3. Cost per case.

Block contracts cover a 'block' of services whereas cost and volume contracts cover an agreed number of cases at a specified price for each case

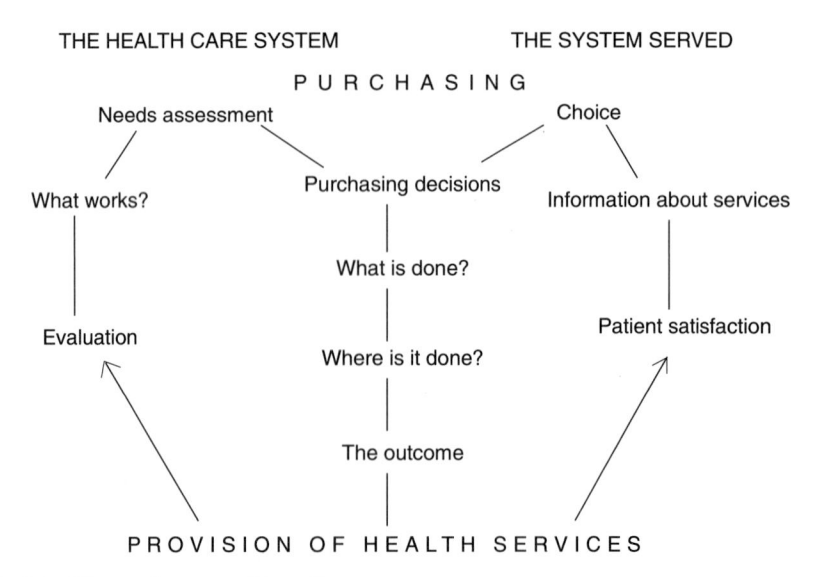

Fig. 3.3 The purchaser-provider split.

```
PURCHASERS          District Health Authorities
                         ╱    │       │    ╲
PROVIDERS          Hospitals  NHS Trusts  Fundholding GPs  Private services
```

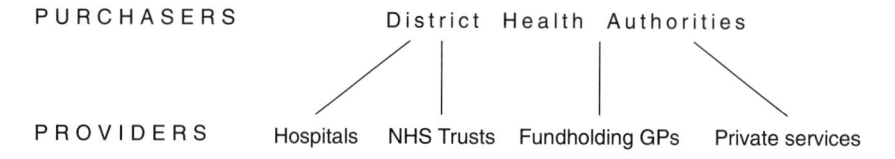

Fig. 3.4 Purchaser–provider split.

with discounts for volume. Cost per case is based on a particular price for a single case.

Currently, the district health authority acts to negotiate these contracts on behalf of GPs. Fundholding practices will negotiate these contracts themselves. It is essential that all GPs take part in these negotiations, either by making their own contracts directly or by making their views and requirements clear to the DHA who will act on their behalf.

The ability to do this has put GPs in a powerful position to influence the quality of care provided for their patients. It has highlighted the importance of particular courses of action being efficient, effective and appropriate. If a hospital does not provide a quick, courteous and competent service then GPs can choose to send their patients elsewhere. This should help to reduce waiting times and improve the service that patients receive when they actually attend hospital.

The system does, however, raise other important issues. What happens to extracontractual referrals — that is, payment by health authorities for treatment by providers with whom there is no contract to purchase care? Health authorities may rightly object to the expensive nature, or dubious value, of patients being treated long distances away when similar treatment is available at lower cost in their own area. However, it is possible that in some ways patient choice will be reduced, as every referral to a specialist centre, or to where a particularly good clinical opinion can be obtained, may now be open to question and refused.

What happens if the health authority exceeds its budget for referrals before the year end? Do they then not allow any further referrals? Do they borrow the money from next year's budget? These questions are unresolved and particularly pertinent as the difficulties in pricing services, with wide area variations, have become apparent.

Practice budgets and fundholding

Just as hospitals now have the opportunity to become NHS trusts, so general practitioners can apply to become fundholders. The current regulations are such that only larger practices, with more than 9000 patients, can do this, although smaller partnerships can band together and negotiate jointly for this purpose. It is likely that these requirements will be altered so that smaller practices can apply in the future.

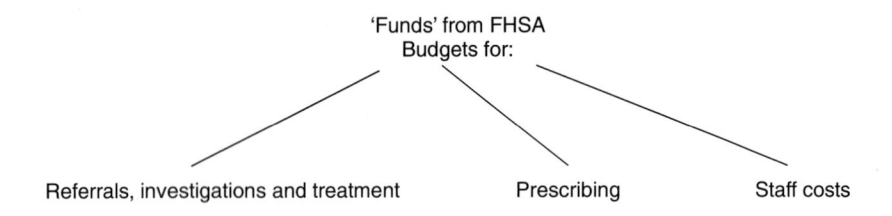

```
                    'Funds' from FHSA
                       Budgets for:
         /                  |                   \
Referrals, investigations    Prescribing         Staff costs
    and treatment
```

Fig. 3.5

Fundholding practices must negotiate annually with their FHSA in order to obtain finance to cover the costs of referrals of patients to hospital, their investigation and treatment. They must also obtain funding for prescribing and employment of staff (Fig. 3.5).

The funding of these different budgets can be transferred so that if one is underspent the saving can be used towards another. For example, if less is spent on prescribing than budgeted for then the savings could be used for extra hospital referrals or to employ more staff.

If the overall budget is underspent, the fundholding practice is allowed to keep a proportion of the savings as long as this extra money is utilised in justifiable improvements to the practice, such as extending premises, buying new equipment and so forth.

Once finance has been obtained, fundholding offers wide scope for purchasing services. Arrangements for referral to hospital have been discussed above, but should it be cheaper or more effective to do so, it is possible to refer outside the NHS. Thus it may be quicker and/or cheaper to arrange for a patient to be seen privately. Also, pathology services may be better provided from a laboratory other than that in the local district general hospital. There is no reason why GPs should not set up their own limited company and provide a pathology service themselves, provided it can be justified in terms of cost and efficiency. This stimulus to competition is intended to ensure that all providers of services make efforts to reduce wastage and inefficiency with the long-term aim of reducing costs or providing a better service for the same cost.

Non-fundholding GPs also have budgets but they do not exercise the same direct control over them as fundholders. Thus they must obtain approval from the FHSA for staff employed at the start of each financial year if they are going to be reimbursed a proportion of the costs. In addition, the practice is set an 'indicative' drug budget, taking into account likely changes in list size, prescribing behaviour and increased costs of the drugs themselves. At the present time there is no penalty for exceeding these agreed limits but it is not clear that this will continue to be the case. Finally, the budget for referrals and hospital treatment is negotiated on their behalf by the district health authority with the hospitals.

In theory, the DHAs are best positioned to negotiate with the provider services because they are acting on behalf of the largest number of GPs and therefore the largest budget. They should thus be able to obtain the largest discounts for bulk purchasing, etc. In reality this may not be the case. Each practice is different, with differing cultural and social class mixes of population, and varying requirements for service provision. The people with the most intimate knowledge of their requirements are therefore the GPs themselves. Thus it may be necessary to be a fundholding practice to ensure the best service possible for the patient.

The basic premise of these systems of financing is open to question. With such a heavy emphasis on efficient use of resources, each decision taken is coloured by its cost implications. Thus, for example, a hospital may decide not to prescribe for outpatients, but rather recommend that patients attend their own GPs surgeries in order to collect their prescriptions. This means that the patients have to pay further trips to the GPs, using up both their own time and that of the practice staff and perhaps the GPs too. If an individual's own GP is not there, either a partner will have to make out the prescription or the patient will have to make yet another trip back to collect it when his/her own doctor has returned. Furthermore, the cost of this prescription has to come out of one budget or another: a cost transferred is not a cost deleted! There may even be a conflict between the hospital and the GP over the drug concerned. If the patient has been recommended a particular treatment by the hospital, it may be no more effective than a cheaper alternative that could be prescribed by the GP, placing the latter in the potentially invidious situation of telling the patient that he or she is going to be prescribed an equivalent because it is *cheaper*. As the hospital is regarded as containing the 'experts' this can lead to conflict between GPs and their patients.

This may be regarded as a trivial example but it nevertheless illustrates the potential pitfalls of a system based on cost. Clearly, doctors must continue to exercise their clinical judgement as to what constitutes the best care for their patients. In doing so they must have regard to the costs of any action taken. While a system based on controlling costs undoubtedly raises the perception for both doctor and patient of just how expensive a particular course of action may be, the emphasis on price may lead to decisions being taken on this basis rather than on purely clinical grounds.

If every decision was clear cut and certain then this would not be an issue. However, general practice is not a straightforward science but is based upon social, cultural, emotional and psychological factors, and knowledge of patients based on their continuing care. For example, most respiratory infections do not require antibiotics, but in some families it is clear that one child always becomes ill (Meyer & Haggerty 1962); in these cases it may be perfectly justifiable to prescribe.

(Thus, deciding to become a fundholding practice has moral and ethical as well as financial implications. If it is possible to improve patient services through assuming direct responsibility for use of funds then this system will be seen as a great step forward for general practice.)

Checklist for trainees

- Is fundholding different to the rest of general practice? If so, why?
- How does a practice reach a decision to become fundholders?
- What is the ethical basis for this decision?
- What moral dilemmas does fundholding present?
- What resources are needed?
- What management skills are required?
- Does it make general practice more accountable?
- Is this system a way of 'aware' general practices making a financial killing?
- If so, at whose expense is it?

DISCUSSION POINT

Fundholding

As the administrative requirements for fundholding are so large, it is likely that this will not be a practical option for small practices. Even though some financial help is available to take the necessary administrative actions to become fundholding, most single-handed GPs or smaller groups will have to pool resources or amalgamate. Should fundholding be shown to be so much better able to provide comprehensive patient services then it is possible that smaller practices would not survive.

— Should all single-handed practices now merge with their larger neighbours in order to take advantage of the potential benefits of fundholding?

— What, if anything, would be lost by so doing?

Prescribing

The Indicative Prescribing Scheme was introduced with the 1990 Contract and took effect in April 1991. It was stated clearly at the time that the objective of the new arrangement was to place downward pressure on drugs expenditure. The key points were that 'the indicative prescribing scheme is truly indicative and will not in any way infringe the rights of medical practitioners to prescribe all the drugs which their patients need', and 'every patient cared for by a general practitioner will always be able to get the drugs that he or she needs, including high-cost medicines, for as long as they are needed'.

The Indicative Prescribing Amount (IPA)

The Indicative Prescribing Amount is the amount of money that each practice is expected to spend on drugs in the coming year. This amount is calculated from a set formula determined by the Department of Health. This is based on the number of prescribing units for each GP. A prescribing unit is any patient registered on a GP's list, but with a weighting factor for patients over the age of 75. This is multiplied by the cost per prescribing unit and an 'uplift' factor. The 'uplift' factor is intended to account for inflation. The cost per prescribing unit is based on historical information, i.e. what the practice spent on drugs and appliances two years ago.

These calculations do not take into account the practice's social and demographic characteristics, and the IPAs are expected to be varied by the practice in negotiation with the FHSA medical or pharmaceutical advisor, who sets the amounts. Factors like the practice taking on a residential home for the elderly could increase the cost of prescribing considerably. Similarly, cost shifting of expensive items such as drugs for infertility treatment or renal dialysis from hospitals to general practice could dramatically inflate the general practice drugs bill.

At the time of writing, IPAs are indicative amounts, and not budgets in the true sense. The consequences for overspending are unclear, although the implications for fundholding practices may be easier to understand.

Prescribing Analysis and Cost (PACT)

The Prescription Pricing Authority (PPA) produces quarterly reports on prescribing by GPs (PACT) at three levels of aggregation. *Level 1* is a simple quarterly analysis of overall prescribing for a practice based on cost, number of items prescribed, cost per item, and the proportion of drugs prescribed in the generic form. Information based on the six leading chapters in the British National Formulary and information for individual doctors are also provided. PACT level 1 is automatically sent to all GPs. *Level 2* focuses on cost with more detailed analysis of the most expensive section. *Level 3* is the most comprehensive, giving more details of the information provided in levels 1 and 2. Details about specific drugs in each category are supplied. For example, it would be possible to see the actual range of antibiotics that is prescribed. PACT levels 2 and 3 are available on request for each practice. Aggregate reports are produced for each FHSA area and nationally using the same format. This enables doctors to use the FHSA and national figures for comparison. The Department of Health has published a guide to audit and research using PACT data (Harris et al 1990).

Any conclusions about the 'appropriateness' of prescribing based on PACT data should be drawn with caution. Principals in a group practice may use each other's prescription forms, and trainees may use the trainer's or other partners' forms so that the individual doctor's prescribing costs may be inaccurate. Furthermore, cost alone is not an indicator of the appropriateness of prescribing; the issue of quality in prescribing is complex and difficult to define. GPs' prescribing patterns are influenced by a variety of factors. These broadly divide into five groups (Hemminki 1975):

- Medical education
- Advertising
- Influence of colleagues
- Expectations of patients and society
- Doctor and practice characteristics.

Education It has been suggested that education positively influences the quality of prescribing, although the studies concerned do not define what is meant by quality and merely show that higher education qualifications are associated with less prescribing of drugs of any kind.

Advertising The contribution of advertising by the drug industry to prescribing is controversial, particularly in terms of accurate and objective information. But pharmaceutical industry promotion does influence prescribing. This is borne out by a study in Northern Ireland (Wyatt et al 1990) in which it was found that there was a sudden but dramatic increase in the prescribing of pivampicillin in 1987–8, after several years of declining use, which corresponded with concerted local promotion by the manufacturers.

Influence of colleagues Many reported studies state that doctors find their colleagues an important source of prescribing information, but this effect is usually secondary to other factors such as education and advertising.

Expectations of patients and society Little work has been done on the effect of patients' demands on prescribing but we are all aware of situations where patients' expectations have influenced our decision to prescribe. Doctors have responsibility to educate about appropriate use of medication but this is a long-term process and is affected by other influences such as advertising and the media.

Doctor and practice characteristics There is evidence that smaller list size and greater time spent with patients are associated with increased prescribing. A plausible explanation is that the doctors with smaller lists can spend more time with each patient and are therefore likely to find out about more conditions that require treatment. This is shown in a study of prescribing patterns in general practice in Northern Ireland, comparing high- and low-cost prescribers (McGavock 1988). It seems possible, therefore, that low-cost prescribing may, in some cases, reflect under-diagnosis and under-treatment as opposed to heightened efficiency.

Summary A review of the factors that affect doctors' prescribing suggests that not only medical factors, but also the pharmaceutical industry, patients, society and the characteristics of the doctors are all major influences. The Indicative Prescribing Scheme focuses on the cost of prescribing without taking any of these factors into account. At the same time 'appropriate' or 'quality' prescribing has not been defined. We may well feel that the doctor who spends more time with patients, unravelling their problems is a better doctor, but his/her prescribing may be more costly.

Pay for general practitioners

Most GPs would like to earn more and believe that the role of general practice within the NHS is undervalued (BMA 1992). You may feel that if you work hard that you will achieve a high income. This sounds a reasonable belief but, in fact, there is a large variation in earnings between various GPs, with some very hard-working practices being comparatively low-income generators. Why should this be so?

In order to consider these differences it is essential to understand the basis of remuneration in general practice; this is the contract that GPs have with the FHSA. Payment is made for services provided (see the list of forms in Appendix II) and allows for considerable discretion in how practices are run and, consequently, how much individual GPs earn. This freedom to practise in different ways, providing that the stipulations of the contract are carried out, enables GPs to have an *independent contractor status.*

GPs are paid by the NHS for the services that they provide. These payments should cover expenses and also provide a net income. Some expenses, such as surgery rent, are reimbursed directly. Other expenses are paid indirectly through fees and allowances (see Appendix III). These are comprehensively listed in the 'Red Book' (National Health Service General Medical Services 1990). GPs may also receive additional private income.

The *average* remuneration that GPs should receive is recommended to the Government by an independent Doctors' and Dentists' Review Body. This recommendation can be (and has been) modified or rejected by the Government, although this should only happen for compelling reasons. A sample of GPs is asked to submit accounts to the Review Body; consequently it is important that all expenses incurred are shown. If expenses are matched against income and 'netted off' this will reduce the overall funding to general practice.

It is important, therefore, that GPs are able to interpret a simple balance sheet (see Fig. 3.6), both to monitor their own financial performance and for the profession as a whole.

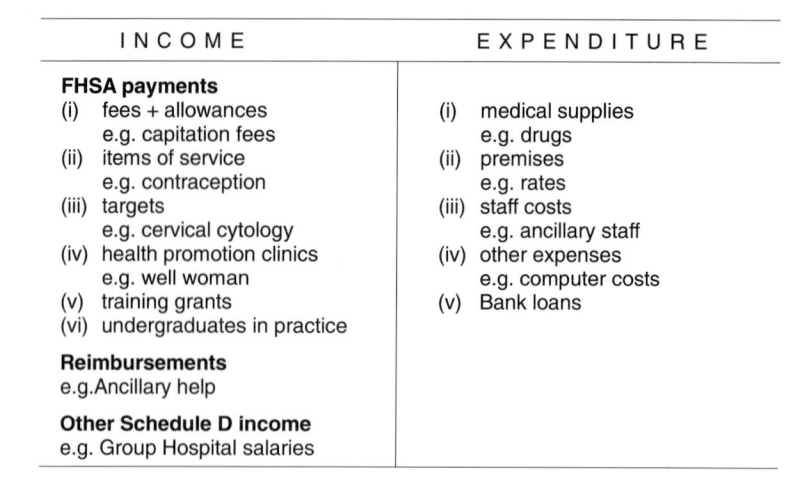

INCOME	EXPENDITURE

FHSA payments
(i) fees + allowances
    e.g. capitation fees
(ii) items of service
    e.g. contraception
(iii) targets
    e.g. cervical cytology
(iv) health promotion clinics
    e.g. well woman
(v) training grants
(vi) undergraduates in practice
Reimbursements
e.g. Ancillary help
Other Schedule D income
e.g. Group Hospital salaries
	(i) medical supplies
	    e.g. drugs
	(ii) premises
	    e.g. rates
	(iii) staff costs
	    e.g. ancillary staff
	(iv) other expenses
	    e.g. computer costs
	(v) Bank loans

Fig. 3.6 A simple balance sheet. (Fees and allowances are intended to make up, on average, 61% of income. The major expense in most practices is staff costs.)

In order to maximise your income it is necessary to keep a tight rein on expenses and to ensure that all fees are claimed and targets met (see specimen balance sheet — Appendix IV).

Expenses

The largest item on the expenses side of most partnership balance sheets is likely to be staff costs (see Appendix IV). Much of this cost is reimbursable and will also appear in the receipts column, dependent on approval for these staff being obtained from the FHSA. As not all the staff salaries will be refunded there may be a substantial net outflow of money. Clearly, it is difficult to practice efficiently without adequate staff and it would not be possible to reach all targets or claim all fees without ancillary help and support. Furthermore, employing other people allows GPs to get on with practising medicine — or taking time off! Thus sensible employment of staff facilitates good use of medical resources as well as being a compromise between costs and income.

Other costs, such as rent or rates, may be directly reimbursed and will not have a major impact on net income (unless they are not claimed for!).

There are numerous items which may not of themselves be large sums but which, added together, can have a substantial effect on the overall accounts. These include costs such as postage and stationery. Simple measures can substantially reduce such costs. It is, for example, sensible to use postage-paid envelopes rather than stamped addressed envelopes when sending out mail requesting a reply: this will save on unused stamps. Telephone bills can be reduced by making non-urgent phone calls after peak time.

Receipts

These can be divided into the following major areas:

1. Capitation fees
2. Items of service
3. Target payments
4. Health promotion
5. Additional sources of income.

It is probably easier to maximise income by concentrating most effort on increasing receipts. The major influence on this is the number of patients on the practice list: the larger the list size, the greater practice income is likely to be.

1. Capitation fees Capitation fees account for nearly two thirds of intended FHSA receipts. This high proportion is intended to create competition between practices for patients and thus improve the quality and number of services available to the patients. It is essential to realise that the capitation fees paid to a GP depend on the number of patients that the FHSA believes, from the registration data, that the GP is looking after. Thus, if a practice has 5000 patients on its list but the FHSA list is only 4000, the capitation fees will be paid for the lower figure. This can amount to a considerable amount of money; it is necessary for GPs to ensure that their lists and those of the FHSA match up as closely as possible. Furthermore, if a GP provides an item of service to a patient, e.g. contraceptive services, then he/she will not be paid for this unless that patient is also on the FHSA list.

Of course these discrepancies can work to a GP's advantage. If a patient has left the list but not yet registered elsewhere, or if a patient has emigrated, then the GP will still be paid as long as that patient is still on the FHSA list. On the whole these differences tend to even out because, if a patient has moved, the GP in the new area will not be paid for this patient until the latter registers.

2. Items of service There are several items of service for which a fee is payable such as contraceptive services, vaccinations, night visits, maternity medical services, etc.

Each item is paid under certain specified circumstances and must be claimed on a specific form. For instance, a night visit fee is payable where a request is made and a visit is performed between 10 p.m. and 8 a.m. The higher rate is payable where a visit is made by a doctor in the same group practice, including the trainee, or by a doctor in a local rota of no more than 10, and a lower rate is paid when a commercial deputising service is used. The claim for payment is made using form FP81 (see Appendix II).

It is important that an efficient system of completing and sending off claim forms is set up as regular monitoring of these can allow income to be maximised. This principle applies whichever item is concerned. A good example may be contraceptive services. Ordinary contraceptive services (which in most circumstances means supplying the oral contraceptive pill) attracts a fee of £12.75 and is claimable on form FP1001. In a practice of 10 000 patients there will be about 2000 women for whom contraceptive services potentially may be required. This is possible annual income of £25 500. An efficient practice might claim for 80% of this (about £20 000) whereas a disorganised one might reach about one third of the potential (about £8000). This represents a difference in income for these hypothetical practices *for this one item alone* of £12 000!

If this is applied across the board, i.e. to capitation, targets, health promotion clinics and so forth, then it is possible for two practices with identical list sizes to have huge differences, perhaps more than £100 000, in income receivable.

3. Target payments Target payments are made for childhood immunisations and cervical smears. These were introduced as an incentive to GPs to see that as many women as possible in the target age range had a recent cervical smear and that the figures for childhood immunisation were improved.

The percentages are calculated on a quarterly basis and the regulations governing these targets are quite complex. For childhood immunisation, for example, for 2-year-olds and 5-year-olds respectively, the regulations stipulate that payment will be made for achieving 70% at the lower level and 90% at the upper level for *completed* courses of immunisation. Once a target has been attained then the figure payable is based on the number of courses completed by doctors as part of general medical services as opposed to those completed elsewhere, such as abroad, privately or at health authority clinics (Chisholm 1990).

4. Health promotion At present the FHSA will pay a fee for clinics performed in general practice provided that a protocol is agreed beforehand. These can provide a considerable source of income to a practice. There is one clinic per GP per week on average. For a four-doctor practice this would bring in nearly £10 000 per annum. In an enthusiastic practice doing three clinics per GP per week, the figure would be nearly £30 000. Even after allowing for cost — nursing, doctor and receptionist time, use of room and equipment, etc. — this still represents a substantial sum of money.

The organisation of health promotion into bands, requiring target groups to have a number of health parameters recorded, means that this system of payment will be abandoned. Instead, payment will be made on agreed objectives — both nationally, and locally with the FHSA — in much the same way that remuneration is now made for reaching cervical cytology or immunisation targets. The exact figures for the various bands have not yet been announced but it seems likely that there will be no new money, and that all payments will be a distribution of what is already present in the pool.

5. *Additional sources of income* There are several other potential sources of income:

- Private income — e.g. private patients, insurance medicals
- Extra work — e.g. course organiser, hospital sessions
- Trainee
- Education — PGEA.

On the whole, their contribution to practice finances forms a small percentage and does not compare with the monies receivable through general medical services. Nevertheless, if time is spent concentrating on these activities then they can make a significant contribution to the financial health of the practice.

All these items involve time and work before they bring in extra income. Nevertheless, the amount of effort expended need not be very large and may simply involve claiming for work being done anyway. There is a fee payable by the county council, for example, for completing a disabled driver's form, i.e. the red badge scheme. These have to be completed anyway; claiming for one per week will bring in nearly £1000 per annum. Attending a suitably approved 5-day educational course once a year will attract a payment of more than £2000.

Thus, if all these activities are looked at closely, and work being done is claimed for, a practice can considerably improve its financial performance.

Remuneration — the future?

The whole basis of remuneration can seem somewhat arbitrary with payments being made simply for the number of years worked in general practice (seniority awards) and percentages seemingly plucked out of the air for target payments. Deprivation payments can be used as an example of this (see below).

The whole structure of payment in general practice can thus be seen as complicated and cumbersome and, in some instances, distinctly unfair. This has led to considerable debate as to the future organisation of general practice remuneration.

There has been some discussion of a move towards a salaried service, on much the same basis as hospital work. Indeed, some GPs are already salaried, e.g. Assistants, Trainees, Associates, etc. However, the majority of GPs are, to date, opposed to such a move.

The major advantage of independent contractor status is that it allows individual GPs independence and freedom in the way their practices are run. Improvements and changes can be introduced without going through bureaucratic tangles. The complicated system of payment and remuneration may be seen as a small price to pay for the scope it allows GPs to carry out practice as they see best.

Since the 1990 Contract changes there has been more management control over GPs' work. In addition, the advantages of being self-employed have to be weighed against the financial security of a predictable level of income. There may, therefore, be a greater move towards a salaried service in the future, especially if the freedom of GPs to run their practices as they wish continues to be reduced.

Deprivation payments These were introduced on the basis that some sections of the community were 'deprived' — mostly in terms of income, housing facilities, etc. — and that these people suffered more illness and therefore required more medical care. The payments serve to reward GPs who work in these areas, particularly as targets are difficult to achieve. In addition, it was hoped that this extra money would attract more GPs to work in these mostly unpopular, inner-city areas.

It is, however, open to debate as to whether these payments will improve the quality of care in the areas concerned. The sums involved are large and it may be that these payments act as a disincentive to even *try* and reach target figures by immunising children and performing cervical smears. GPs who are entitled to claim under these regulations could 'take the money and run'! Perhaps this requires a rethink?

DISCUSSION POINT

Deprivation payments

These are based on the concept of a section of the population being socially and financially under-resourced and thus vulnerable to ill-health.

— What is the evidence for this?

— Is there any evidence that increasing medical resources to this population will lead to an improvement in their health?

— Are deprivation payments to general practitioners the best way of improving health in inner-city areas?

Seniority awards

Seniority allowances are paid to GPs who have been registered with the General Medical Council and have served as an unrestricted NHS principal for the required number of years. At present these payments are made in three stages with the first level payable after 11 years registration with the GMC and 7 years as a GP. They are intended to reward GPs for the extra expertise gained over the years in practice.

— what evidence is there that GPs become 'better' at their job as they gain more experience?

— How do you define what is a 'good GP'?

— What other options are available to reward high standards of medical care?

— What are the advantages and drawbacks of a 'merit award' system, as used for hospital consultants?

— Should there be a register of 'good' doctors?

IV. THE 'TRAINEE EFFECT'

Less obvious than the effect a training practice has on a trainee is the impact she or he has upon the practice. This will vary depending on the experience and personality of each trainee. Organisational requirements of a training practice can therefore be divided into those that are standard (see list below), those that depend largely on the characteristics of an individual trainee, and those that are a combination of both. Compulsory training requirements are:

- Notes and letters
- Summaries
- Premises
- Ancillary staff
- Equipment
- Library
- Study leave
- Holidays
- Teaching time
- Half-day release
- Consulting
- Night visits.

Checklist for trainees	
Notes and letters:	Are these in date order, tagged and legible?
Summaries:	Are diagnostic summaries and regular prescriptions clearly recorded?
Premises:	Are these adequate for the size of the practice, well organised and maintained?
Ancillary staff:	Are there sufficient staff for the practice, and are they satisfactorily trained?
Equipment:	Is there modern and functional equipment and is it used?
Library:	Is there one, and does it contain up-to-date textbooks and journals relevant to general practice and postgraduate education?
Study leave:	Is this provided for the trainee?
Teaching:	Is regular, protected time made available for teaching and learning in the practice? Is it of sufficient quality and variety? Is assessment agreed and performed?
Half-day release:	Is attendance at a local half-day release scheme allowed and encouraged?
Consulting:	Are enough surgeries and home visits organised? Is there support in case of difficulties?
Night visits:	When does the trainee participate in the on-call rota? Is there back-up from the trainer or other partners?

In order for a practice to be approved for training it first has to be inspected by the Regional Advisor in General Practice, or one of his/her assistants, to ascertain that it at least attains the minimum required standards. A GP from that practice has to undertake a training course, and be approved, before a trainee can be appointed. Both the practice and the trainer have to undergo periodic reassessment. It is expected that a trainer and the practice will provide excellent opportunities for a trainee to learn and gain experience in general practice without being used as 'an extra pair of hands'. Practice organisation is looked at as an integral part of this and each component is expected to reach a minimum standard.

All these conditions need to be met satisfactorily for a practice to be allowed to continue training. The requirements may alter — e.g. the percentage requirement for notes to be adequately summarised has risen from 20% a few years ago to 80% or more in most regions. These stipulations require time, effort and expenditure by a practice. Putting notes in order needs suitably trained staff to do it. Buying textbooks for the library can cost a lot money. Time used by a trainer to prepare a tutorial could be otherwise spent seeing patients. A trainee may be a luxury that a practice finds hard to afford. Equally, some practices may regard a trainee as an essential stimulus to development. This is a balance that will vary from practice to practice and depends on the characteristics of the organisation and individuals involved (see Table 3.4).

The decision for a practice to become involved in postgraduate training is therefore not one to be taken without a due consideration of the potential problems involved as well as the benefits that may accrue. Nevertheless, the requirements for organisation seem sensible for all practices to aim at, whether or not they are going to be involved in training.

Conclusions

There is a strain between earning a living and doing a good job. It is important to consider family and friends as well as working environment when choosing a practice. There *is* life outside the surgery; Armstrong in

Table 3.4 The trainee: help or hindrance?

Benefits	Disadvantages
Time saved	*Time used*
Surgeries	Teaching preparations
Visits	Tutorials
Night calls	Sitting in, joint visits
Income	*Costs*
Training grant	Books, equipment, premises, courses.
Help	*Hindrance*
Ideas person	Upsets practice routine
Practice development	Safe with patients?

his article on space and time (Armstrong 1985) has noted how general practice has changed over the years, moving from single practitioners working in their own homes to large partnerships sharing on-duty rotas, working from purpose-built premises.

Comparisons of partnerships with marriage or other close and complex relationships are often made. Consequently, learning about the practice in which you work is a way of helping to make life as a GP more understandable, and perhaps help to share the burdens and stresses of other people's expectations. Your own aspirations are important too, but are they realistic? Do the other partners share the same ideals and goals?

The enthusiastic trainee runs the risk of 'burnout' and turning into the disillusioned, careworn GP. Learning to be pragmatic about what can be done, and understanding your own limitations and the limitations of others, will help you to approach the task of changing the way you work in a sensible manner. A consultation with a patient is one in a whole series allowing a gradual picture to emerge of the patient as a unique individual with his or her own problems. In a similar way each practice has developed its own characteristics over a long period and so it may take time to bring about changes in working practices. Understanding how a practice is organised increases the opportunities to influence its further evolution.

General practice is going through an intense period of change, both in the services it is expected to provide and in the way it is financed. It is likely that this will lead to a completely different type of practice in the future, with changing contractual, organisational and financial requirements. It is possible that, in order to offer as wide a range of services as possible, GPs will join together in 'health shops' with opticians, pharmacists, physiotherapists and others. This requires goodwill on behalf of all those concerned, as well as understanding from the patients and financial support from the Government.

The trainee year provides an excellent opportunity to learn how general practice is organised and financed, and how an individual practice functions. A good understanding acquired now should help the trainee through the rest of his or her career.

REFERENCES

Arber S 1987 What is a good GP? British Medical Journal 294: 287–288
Arber S, Sawyer L 1985 The role of the receptionist in General Practice: A 'dragon behind the desk'? Social Science and Medicine 20: 911–921
Armstrong D 1985 Space and time in British general practice. Social Science and Medicine 20: 659–666
Cartwright A 1986 A depressing pursuit of quality. British Medical Journal 292: 1497–1498
Chisholm J 1990 Making sense of the new contract. Radcliffe Medical Press, Oxford.
Copeman J P, Van Swanenberg T D 1988 Practice receptionists: Poorly trained and taken for granted? Journal of the Royal College of General Practitioners 38: 14–16
Department of Health and Social Security 1986 Cumberlege Report. Neighbourhood nursing — a focus for care. Report of the Community Nursing Review. HMSO, London

Department of Health 1989 Terms of service for doctors in general practice, HMSO, London
Harris C, Heywood P, Clayden A 1990 The analysis of prescribing in general practice: a guide to audit and research. HMSO, London
Heath C 1987 What is a good GP? British Medical Journal 294: 415–416
Hemminki E 1975 Review of literature on the factors affecting prescribing. Social Science and Medicine 9: 111–115
Hill P 1991 Purchaser-provider split. Royal College of General Practitioners, Connection, Nov: 12
Iliffe S, Haug U 1991 Out of hours work in general practice. British Medical Journal 302: 1584–1586
McGavock H 1988 Some patterns of prescribing by urban general practitioners. British Medical Journal 296: 900–902
Meyer R J, Haggerty R J 1962 Streptococcal infections in families. Pediatrics 29: 539–549
National Health Service General Medical Services 1990 Statement of fees and allowances payable to General Medical Practitioners in England and Wales. Department of Health, Welsh Office
Pendleton D 1985 In: Sheldon M, Brooke J, Rector A (eds). Decision-making in general practice. Macmillan, London
Pill R, Stott N C H 1982 Concepts of illness causation and responsibility: some preliminary data from a sample of working-class mothers. Social Science and Medicine 16: 43–52
Salisbury C J 1989 How do people choose their doctor? British Medical Journal 299: 608–610
Wyatt T, Passmore C, Morrow N, Reilly P 1990 Antibiotic prescribing: the need for a policy in general practice. British Medical Journal 296: 900–902

FURTHER READING

British Medical Association 1983 Organising a practice. Articles from the British Medical Journal. British Medical Association, London.
Campbell A V, Higgs R 1982 In that case. Medical ethics in everyday practice. Dartman, Longman & Todd, London
Gillon R 1985 Philosophical medical ethics. Wiley, Chichester
General Medical Services Committee 1991 Your choices for the future. British Medical Association, London

APPENDIX I

Specimen job description for receptionist

JOB TITLE: Receptionist
RESPONSIBLE TO: The Partners
AT: Central Surgery
UNDER SUPERVISION OF: Practice Manager
SALARY GRADE:

DUTIES
1. Open premises.
2. Handle general enquiries, explain surgery procedures, make new and follow-up appointments.
3. Hand out prescriptions, referral letters and certificates.
4. Reception and routing of patients on arrival.
5. Take telephone enquiries for appointments.
6. Answer telephone and re-route calls.
7. Make appointments for nurse's clinics.
8. Registration of new patients, follow practice policy.
9. Compile and update lists for surgeries.
10. Give information on inoculations and vaccinations.
11. File prescriptions, referral letters and certificates.
12. Put out information leaflets.
13. Accept specimens.
14. Order reception area stationery.
15. Air and tidy waiting rooms.
16. Tuition of new staff.
17. Cancel surgeries.
18. Leave reception area tidy and ready for incoming colleagues.
19. Leave information regarding unsolved or urgent problems.
20. Any such other duties as agreed with Partners.

APPENDIX II

List of forms

(Based on England and Wales — different forms and fees may apply to Scotland or Northern Ireland although the structure is very similar.)

A. To be completed by doctor

PRESCRIPTIONS

FP10	— Prescriptions.
FP10 COMP	— Prescriptions on computer.

CERTIFICATION

Med 3	— Ordinary medical certificates.
Med 5	— Backdated medical certificates (or where a letter has been received but the patient has not been seen).
Med 6	— Confidential diagnosis to be sent to Regional Medical Officer where only a 'vague' diagnosis has been put on form Med 3 or Med 5
Med 7	— Form to be sent to Regional Medical Officer in confidence asking for a second opinion, e.g. where there may some doubt as to the 'genuine' nature of the illness.
RM2	— Form from District Medical Officer for opinion on patient's capacity to work.
RM8	— Form sent by Regional Medical Officer asking for more details of a patient's illness, e.g. where there has been an extended period of certificated sickness.

REGISTRATION AND RECORDS

FP1	— Application to go on a doctor's list (completed by patient and signed by doctor).
FP7	— Male continuation card.
FP8	— Female continuation card.
FP9	— Summary of treatment card (A for males, B for females).
FP19	— Temporary residents.
FP1011	— Immunisation record card.

CLAIM FORMS

FP 32	— Emergency treatment.
FP 81	— Night visits.
FP 106	— Immediately necessary treatment
FP 82	— Arrest of dental haemorrhage.
FPRF	— Registration fees.
FP/HPC	— Health promotion clinic fees.
FP/MS	— Minor surgery fees.
	Child Health Surveillance fee.

Contraception

FP1001	— Ordinary contraceptive services.
FP1002	— Fitting an intrauterine contraceptive device.
FP1003	— Contraceptive services for visitors.

Maternity care
FP24 — Provision of maternity care.
　　　　Lower fees apply if a doctor is not on the Obstetric List.

Immunisations
FP73 — Vaccinations.

B. To be completed by patient
Mat B1 — Allows woman to claim maternity allowance — to be completed between 26 and 29 weeks.
FW8 — Allows woman to claim free vitamins and prescriptions during pregnancy.
SC1 — Self-certificate and Invalidity Benefit claim form.

APPENDIX III

List of Fees and Allowances
(For comprehensive list please see *Statement of fees and allowances*.)

A. Capitation and allowances
CAPITATION FEES
- Under 65
- 65–74
- 75 plus

FP19 *Temporary residents:*
higher rate — patient in area 16 days–3 months
lower rate — patient in area 1–15 days.

Deprivation payments
High, medium or low levels per patient.

BASIC PRACTICE ALLOWANCE
(A reduced allowance applies where there are less than 1200 patients/GP in the practice.)

SENIORITY ALLOWANCE
Value per GP:
First payment after 7 years as a GP, increasing after a further 7 years to a medium rate, and then to the maximum rate after 21 years as a GP.

RURAL PRACTICE PAYMENTS
Complicated formula based on percentage of patients in a rural area *and* three miles from surgery.

POSTGRADUATE EDUCATION ALLOWANCE

LEAVE PAYMENTS
Payments are available for various absences. These include:
- Locum allowance during sickness
- Confinement allowance
- Prolonged study leave allowance.

B. Items of service e.g. contraception

C. Target payments
There is a formula based on the average number of patients:
- Immunisation for children aged two or less
- Preschool boosters
- Cervical cytology.

D. Clinics

E. Miscellaneous e.g. prescribing
Supply of drugs and appliances:
A complicated formula exists for reimbursement of each prescription based on the basic drug price less an average discount plus a dispensing fee plus on-cost allowance plus VAT allowance.

F. Trainer's grant

APPENDIX IV

Specimen balance sheet
for Doctors Black, White, James, Alderson, Carp, Purcell and Shanahan.

PRACTICE RECEIPTS
for the year ended 30th April 1991

Family Health Services Authority payments
  Fees and other payments for medical services:

	Capitation Fees:		
	Less than 65	154331	
	65–74	23004	
	>75	36246	
	Temporary residents	3269	
	Night visits	15266	
	Maternity fees	10437	
	Cervical cytology target fees	7872	
	Contraceptive services	9871	
	Minor surgery	4860	
	New registration fees	3672	
	Childhood immunisation target fees:		
	2-year-olds	6896	
	5-year-olds	2065	
	Health promotion clinics	5852	
	Vaccination fees	6555	
	Other fees	3731	
			293927
	Seniority, vocational and Postgraduate training	27351	
	Training grants	4984	
			326262
Reimbursements:			
	Drugs	7075	
	Surgery	23500	
	Rates	7600	
	Ancillary help	95465	
	Trainees	27916	
	Computer	1379	
			162935
Other Schedule D income			
	Group hospitals salaries	8573	
	Other miscellaneous fees	18319	
			26892
			516089

PRACTICE EXPENSES
for the year ended 30th April 1991

General revenue			
	Medical Supplies:		
	Drugs and dressings	6089	
	Towels	1351	
	Equipment, replacements and hire	603	
			8043

Premises:
Rates	6171	
Water	757	
Heat and light	1806	
Insurance	1071	
Repairs and renewals	4223	
Cleaning, etc.	4935	
Telephone and radiopaging	3917	
		22880

Staff costs:
Trainees	28550	
Ancillary staff	137836	
Staff advertising and agency fees	39	
		167425

Other expenses:
Postage	556	
Stationery	1965	
Hire and maintenance of office machinery	1966	
Computer leasing interest	2113	
Computer running expenses	5750	
Medical committee expenses	969	
Medical course fees	2222	
Accountancy and professional services	1034	
Bank charges and overdraft interest	2054	
Bank loan interest	1363	
Sundry expenses	2320	
		21312
		219660

Other payments
Bank loan capital repayments	7149	
Purchases of computer and equipment	2404	
		9553
		229213

TOTAL PRACTICE RECEIPTS	516089
TOTAL PRACTICE EXPENSES	229213
NET PRACTICE INCOME	286876

(for seven partners where the income is divisible equally, this results in a profit share per partner of £40 982)

4. Communication in practice

Richard A. Savage

INTRODUCTION

Communication is the central process of general practice. Clinical competence is, of course, an essential basis for practice, but the skilled GP is first and foremost a skilled communicator. Our working life revolves around communication not just with patients but also with colleagues, staff and a wide variety of outside agencies. It is failure in communication rather than technical error which is the cause of most medical accidents and complaints against doctors.

Doctors' skills in communication have been shown to affect:

- The adequacy of their clinical interviews
- Patient compliance
- Patient recall of advice
- Patient satisfaction
- The impact of potentially distressing procedures
- The ability to detect emotional distress
- The doctor's job satisfaction and stress levels.

This chapter will examine mainly what goes on when doctors communicate with patients in the consultation. This may take place in the traditional setting of the doctor's surgery or it may be in patients' homes, over the telephone or sometimes on a hospital ward. We shall examine the three main elements of the consultation: the doctor, the patient and the setting. Some aspects of consultation theory and some specific communication skills will also be considered.

Some special types of consultation which frequently cause anxiety for trainees are discussed. These are breaking news, talking to angry patients and consulting by telephone.

The second part of the chapter considers some issues outside the consultation. These are trainee-trainer communication, practice team communication and writing hospital referrals.

THE CONSULTATION

Trainees arriving in general practice for the first time often do not think of their previous dealings with patients as consultations. Words like 'clerking', 'admitting', or simply 'seeing' are used to describe their clinical interactions. In spite of the use of different words you have been developing consultation skills throughout your medical career. There are, however, important differences between the consultation process in general practice and the direct history-taking model which is usually employed in hospital medicine. These differences increase with the time you spend in the practice as you get to know your patients better and so less needs to be actually said at each meeting before the immediately relevant communication takes place. The ongoing relationship which GPs develop with their patients can compensate for the shorter consultation time available in general practice.

The doctor and the consultation

As doctors we are taught to make decisions in order to cope with a variety of medical conditions. Our training to some extent suppresses natural personal reactions to severe illness and distress in order to deal with the job of making a diagnosis and delivering necessary treatment. General practice is often concerned with self-limiting or chronic medical problems that also have psychological and social dimensions. The general practitioner needs an expanding view of the patient's problems; this contrasts with the focused view of the specialist. The greater scope of possibilities facing the general practitioner brings uncertainty which feels different from the confidence of knowing a lot about a defined area. It is not possible to know everything in general practice.

Doctors are taught to recognise what they know. Trainees entering the almost infinite realm of general practice need a new skill — that of recognising what they don't know. They have to learn how to cope with uncertainty and ignorance while providing effective patient care. This requires confidence and support.

Uncertainty is helped by:

- Comprehensive medical knowledge. Diagnosing or excluding medical conditions as a cause of symptoms clears the way to explore other possibilities for the patient's 'dis-ease' when appropriate.
- Discovering who is the best person to ask when you don't know.
- Awareness of the self-limiting nature of many conditions, thus freeing you, when necessary, to take on a supportive rather than curative role.
- Seeing the problem from the patient's point of view.

When conventional medicine cannot provide a solution it is often helpful to suspend medical 'objectivity' in order to explore the patient's beliefs and values. Some doctors fear engaging with patient in this way. This fear may stem from lack of respect for the patient's view, the potential loss of control of the consultation or the onus of sharing an emotional burden that the patient might reveal. Yet this can save time and lead to more appropriate management.

Being interested, listening and getting appropriately involved, takes time but saves time in the end.

Doctors often undervalue their uniqueness as people. Personality is an important therapeutic tool. Experience of life equips the doctor with resources that can provide understanding and sympathy for patient dilemmas. Understanding the patient's experience enhances empathy.

Influences on the doctor's communication skills	
• Personality	• Working conditions
• Background	• Patients
• General education	• Administrators
• Medical teachers	• Government
• Other health workers	• Press
• Workload	• Society

Doctors' understanding of their role as general practitioners is similarly influenced. They may feel they are there to be useful, wanted, praised, revered or judgemental, and their perceived role alters their communication style. Doctors may have other aims that can profoundly affect communication style, for example, to remove the patient from the consultation as quickly as possible or to generate as much income from the consultation as possible.

Doctors' communication skills develop by watching their teachers, a process called 'modelling'. The behaviour of patients, contact with others, the interaction of the medical bureaucracy with the Government and the press all affect doctors' image of themselves and their expectations about how patients and others should behave and communicate.

You can monitor the development of communication skills by, for example, reviewing audio or videotaped consultations. These techniques are more effective when done with a trusted peer, a mentor or in the secure atmosphere of a supportive small group. It is important to start monitoring as early as possible in the trainee year as communication styles develop quickly and may become fixed early in the general practitioner's development.

Role play of a consultation is another powerful method of exploring communication and can allow the doctor to experience what it is like to be the patient. In this way you can discover, for example, how it feels to be the recipient of bad news or to be angry about treatment received.

Communication style

Communication style develops early, check it out by:
- Recording your consultations
- Sitting in on other doctors' consultations
- Having others sit with you during surgeries
- Discussing audio/videotaped consultations with others
- Keeping your videos over the year to observe change
- Role play.

It is not necessary to enter psychotherapy in order to be a good general practitioner but awareness of the influence of the relatively fixed aspects of communication style can allow small adjustments that make a big difference to communication. For example: 'what is wrong?' may elicit different information from 'what do you think is wrong?'.

It is very important that you feel 'happy in your skin', a West Indian expression describing feeling good about yourself. Doctors need to be in touch with different aspects of their personality and prejudices and to come to terms with their shortcomings so they feel 'good enough' about themselves. There will then be enough self-confidence to cope with the uncertainties and challenges that general practice poses.

The ability to admit ignorance to yourself and, when appropriate, to the patient, is an essential communication skill. General practitioners need to discover their personal and professional limitations. This needs to be done sensitively and with caution. It is not professional to off-load personal problems, neither should the doctor's powerful position in the relationship be exploited. The doctor should never remove hope or support from the relationship. Developing self-awareness will guard against such abuses and allow sensitive communication during the consultation.

Developing self-awareness

- What are my strengths and weaknesses?
- Am I able to discover my limitations?
- Can I share my limitations with patients when appropriate?
- Am I secure enough to admit to myself when I'm wrong?

The doctor's tasks in the consultation

Stott & Davies (1979) described four areas which can be explored each time a patient consults. Each of these areas represents a communication task.

A. Management of presenting problems Establish the immediate problem or issue. Is the patient suffering from a definable disease? Is it serious? How best can it be treated and by whom?

B. Modification of help-seeking behaviours This is an area of health education: explaining to the patient, for example, the natural history of a minor illness and how they might manage similar problems in the future.

C. Management of continuing problems How is any previous or chronic condition progressing? How well is it controlled?

D. Opportunistic health promotion This is the area of prevention. Is the patient due, for example, for vaccinations or screening procedures?

A fifth area needs to be explored, and that is 'what is the patient's agenda?' i.e. why have they come now, what is really worrying them, and what do they hope I can do for them?

This is usually too much for a 10-minute consultation so the doctor copes by selecting the most important areas. Selection is aided by intuition refined by the skill of 'taking the main chance' by exploring the most likely possibility early in the consultation. General practitioners often tend to make a provisional diagnosis too early in the consultation, so it will help you to listen with an open mind for longer than you might assume is necessary.

It is possible to 'tune in' to patients at an intuitive level to obtain valuable information. Some examples of these subconscious thoughts are: the prickly feeling at the back of the neck when facing a mentally disturbed person, the expression that suggests recently altered mood or health, the transmitted 'feeling' of hostility or care, indifference or concern, panic or confidence, anger or approval, especially if it is inconsistent with what is being said. Intuition can be refined to alert the doctor to new or different problems, but it should be carefully checked and confirmed. It is not enough to take action on intuition alone.

Summary: the doctor and the consultation

The trainee year provides a chance for you to gain insight into your personality and how it interacts with others. It allows the acquisition and reorganisation of medical knowledge to meet the needs of the practice population and allows for the admission of ignorance and uncertainty when appropriate.

Discussion with other trainees exposes differences in approach to general practice problems. Analysis of videotaped consultations shows a different self perception while role play places you in the patient's position to give valuable insights. All these experiences and more give the chance for increased self-awareness that allows the examination of the role of personal experience in the formation of views and attitudes. It gives the chance to experience being part of the patient's life as well as being a medical technician. It offers the chance to explore and refine communication skills to enhance these tasks.

The patient and the consultation

Patients, like doctors, are affected by their personal experience on the journey to the consultation. Many complex influences contribute to a non-professional or lay medical training. Patients have a unique experience of life that influences their views about doctors, illness and its outcome.

A 45-year-old hypertensive man whose father died suddenly of a myocardial infarct was a heavy smoker who resisted health education advice because he assumed the same fate inevitably awaited him. When it was pointed out that he could not count on this assumption he stopped smoking. He had not thought of the consequences of, for example, chronic obstructive airways disease or stroke, whereby he might become dependent on others.

Cultural influences, religious beliefs, dependency on others or stress may influence the meaning ascribed to a symptom. Zborowsky's study of response to pain (1952) showed that Americans of Italian extraction would not be satisfied with their doctor until the pain had been removed because the actual pain sensation caused stress. While it was not manly to complain of pain at home, expression of pain in hospital was acceptable. They also assumed that good medical care would be delivered to cure their symptoms. Jewish people were more concerned with the meaning of the pain and the possible consequences not only for themselves but for their families. Successful management included an explanation of the pain and its implications. They were sceptical of medical care offered, a possible second opinion might be sought and symptoms might be manipulated to ensure that they obtained what they saw as the best medical care. The 'Old American' was more stoical. These patients would attempt to define the pain, underplay symptoms and adopt a detached view. By so doing they would seek approval of the doctor.

Patients try alternative ways of coping before visiting the doctor, for example:

- carrying on as usual and ignoring the symptom
- setting a time limit for its resolution before seeking help
- seeking the advice of trusted friends or relatives
- self medication
- attending an alternative or traditional healer.

Lay expert knowledge acquired in this way influences behaviour, communication and compliance.

Social setting also influences symptom perception: a rugby player may be unaware of an injury until after the game is over while a similar assault in a street may produce instant disability and prolonged psychological trauma. A person caring for a dying relative may not become aware of weight loss or fatigue that heralds the onset of serious disease in him or herself.

Personal experience of visiting general practitioners and hospitals influences how the doctor is seen:

- as an expert with highly developed technical skills who provides treatment
- as an understanding, sympathetic, reassuring figure that smooths the transition from health to sickness and back again
- an idiosyncratic interpretation that ranges through technician, friend, father-figure, faith-healer, loved one.

Similarly, patients have expectations about how the doctor ought to communicate:

- by listening (or ignoring)
- by paying attention (or being busy and distracted)
- by valuing (or being dismissive)
- by helping (or being ineffectual or harmful)
- by appropriate shouldering of responsibility (or over- or under-involvement).

Patients make decisions about how to behave towards the doctor. They may:

- cooperate fully
- withhold or distort information
- hand responsibility to the doctor or continue to be in control
- accept or disregard advice
- seek other opinions or methods of treatment or be passive and fatalistic
- attribute improvement to the doctor's skill or blame the doctor for unwanted outcomes.

If you start to understand the patient's point of view, you are more likely to develop appropriate communication skills.

The separate agendas of doctor and patient in the consultation

Communication may fail completely if the doctor doesn't start from the patient's concerns and view of the problem. You are challenged to attend to two agendas: to be highly medically skilled and a good problem solver and to understand the patient's view (Table 4.1).

The doctor's agenda is reflected in the acronym 'SOAP' (*s*ymptom, *o*bjective, *a*ssessment, *p*lan) that can be used to structure the written record

Table 4.1 Agendas

Doctor	Patient
What is wrong?	Why me?
How can it be fixed?	Why now?
Diagnose or exclude disease	What has caused it?
Minimise medical error	What could happen to me?
Take the 'main chance'	What might the doctor do?
Take chosen action	What does this mean to me?

of the consultation. This can be made more patient-centred by using a new acronym 'SWEAT'. Devised by a South London trainee, 'SWEAT' provides headings as follows:

- *S*ymptom presented
- *W*hat does this mean to the patient (and all the other 'w's in the patient's agenda listed in the right-hand column of Table 4.1)
- *E*xamination
- *A*ssessment
- *T*reatment.

Summary: the patient and the consultation

- Patients are lay medical experts.
- Life experience, culture and social influences inform the patient in identifying and interpreting symptoms.
- There is a rich source of lay medical expertise treatment and coping mechanisms.
- The medical profession influences lay ideas about illness.
- General practitioners are influenced by lay ideas about illness.
- The patient's sense of personal control influences decisions made about symptoms and behaviours affecting health.
- Doctors and patients may have different agendas in the consultation.

The setting of the consultation

How the practice organises contact with patients gives important messages and can affect the consultation. Arranging to see the doctor can be a complicated process. Appointment systems, inefficient telephone switchboards and unhelpful staff can all be adverse influences on communication in the consultation ('I felt like hitting that rude receptionist who said I couldn't see you, who does she think she is?'). Patients who have had to wait a long time may wish to discuss practice organisation rather than their symptoms ('There were lots of people who arrived after me that were seen by the other doctor before me ... why did that lady get seen straight away when I have been waiting forty minutes?'). Others, glad to have breached the practice defence albeit one hour late, proceed to disclose every possible source of ill-health that might threaten in the foreseeable future in order to minimise the chances of having to make another appointment.

These problems can be minimised by:

- a welcoming reception area
- flexible appointment systems
- sympathetic, efficient, highly-trained and courteous staff
- an efficient switchboard professionally handled
- enough space in the waiting area (crowding makes violence more likely)
- when running late: giving updates on waiting times at frequent intervals and apologising to patients for unavoidable delays
- a quiet side room to defuse altercations and to place ill or upset patient
- simple, clear public notices and instructions
- specific times when a doctor is available by telephone.

Distance travelled to see the doctor is also an important factor in doctor availability and may influence mode of communication. It may be easier to phone or ask for a home visit than attempt to travel long distances to the surgery.

When the patient finally arrives in the doctor's room, this too has an effect on the consultation process. The consulting room is the doctor's 'home territory'. Its layout and decoration reflect the doctor's personality and approach to work. A private setting for the doctor-patient relationship is formed in which the doctor is most likely to feel relaxed, confident and in control. The way the consulting room is organised and decorated gives the patient important messages about what to expect and how to behave.

The room instantly tells the patient something about who the doctor is and how available they are. The position of the desk, the height and comfort of the doctor's and patient's chairs, lighting, photographs and pictures create a unique atmosphere. Effective transfer of information is most likely to occur when doctor and patient sit on the same side of the desk, facing each other. Using the desk as a barrier by sitting opposite each other will almost certainly reduce the flow of information.

A hard uncomfortable chair that is about to collapse and that is lower than the doctor's is not going to make the patient feel at ease. Photographs of the doctor's spouse, partner, friends and family discretely displayed can give the patient important information about the doctor's personal life, as can drawings by family members. Among other things this helps the patient to avoid misinterpreting professional care as seeking a more intimate relationship than was intended. Lighting that mimics an interrogation centre is obviously not helpful. An uncluttered desk might give the impression that time and attention are easily available. A discrete telephone bell avoids startling nervous patients and some doctors may in fact advise staff that they should not be interrupted by the telephone while consulting unless it is absolutely essential.

Much is made of doctors' dress. The literature on patient preference favours sober ties, suits and dresses. How much this reflects patients conditioning through habitual exposure to a conservatively-dressed profession is hard to say. Certainly patients in middle-class areas express stronger opinions on this subject than those in inner-city areas.

Summary: the setting of the consultation

Much can be done to facilitate effective communication between doctor and patient before they meet. Physical access and communication, either by telephone or at the reception desk, are an important start. Monitoring appointment systems, open access surgeries, and providing information about waiting times to see the doctor will reduce friction. A comfortable waiting area is desirable. A suitably dressed doctor sitting in a sympathetically organised and lit room with minimal chance of interruption is highly desirable.

The theory of the consultation

What really happens in the consultation?

The literature is strong on rhetoric about how doctors and patients should communicate and behave, but valid evidence to back such claims is harder to come by as it is a difficult area to research. Some observations made have not always been what doctors have wanted to hear about themselves.

Michael Balint in 1957 provided the insight that a doctor's personality interacts with medical training to produce a unique way of dealing with patients. He observed that doctors shy away from examining themselves as people in their performance as doctors so that a fixed style of behaviour towards patients is developed. This 'apostolic function', as he called it, also embodies doctors' beliefs about how patients should behave when ill, how patients should behave with doctors and the sorts of behaviours that patients should adopt in order to cooperate to try to get better. Balint recognised the powerful therapeutic effect of doctors as people, separate from the treatments they offer, and he coined the phrase 'drug doctor' to emphasise this point.

Byrne & Long's 1976 study of general practitioners' audiotaped consultations identified two other influences: the repetitive activity of the consultation and the severe time constraints under which the consultation takes place. They thought that these influences also contributed to a fixed style of behaviour developed by doctors to cope with most problems most of the time. They described a continuum of consulting style which varies from 'doctor-centred' to 'patient-centred'. In the highly doctor-centred consultation, the doctor dominates the interview using direct, closed questions, rejecting the patient's ideas and evading their questions. In the patient-centred interview, the doctor uses such methods as open questions, active listening, challenging and reflecting in order to allow the patient to express themselves in their own way. Byrne & Long also made another, often overlooked observation, that the communication style used by a doctor to elicit information and make a diagnosis may differ from the style used to give advice and treatment.

Other researchers have shown that time constraints alter the amount and content of what is discussed in the consultation. Longer consultations (more than eight minutes) significantly improve patient satisfaction with the consultation and communication, especially if the patient's problem has a major psychological component. Longer consultations allow patients to ask more questions, and doctors to give more explanation, do more health promotion and carry out more disease prevention measures. Treatment subsequently involves less prescribing of medication and patients are less likely to return for the same or other conditions in the following four weeks.

Recently it has been suggested that consultation length is so important that it can be used as a proxy measure of quality of general practice care.

Pendleton et al (1984) influenced doctors' thinking by suggesting that a sharing style can address patients' ideas about their illness so that they will be more likely to be satisfied with their general practitioner and comply with treatment. Seven communication tasks are defined:

1. To define the reasons for the patient's attendance
2. To consider other problems
3. To choose with the patient an appropriate action for each problem
4. To achieve a shared understanding of the problems with the patient
5. To involve the patient in management and sharing of responsibility
6. To use time and resources appropriately
7. To establish and maintain a relationship with the patient that will help achieve the above tasks.

This approach is hampered by the time constraints of an NHS consultation and does not pay attention to the doctor's needs. The doctor usually attends to what is thought to be the main problem first; other problems are then addressed but it may be necessary to postpone dealing with a problem, if there is not enough time. The more there is to do, the less thoroughly each task is handled. A litany of symptoms may suggest an unrelated problem such as anxiety or depression. Occasionally a patient will test the doctor with a minor symptom and only if it is dealt with adequately will then risk presenting the main problem. Sometimes the most important and revealing statements are made just as the patient is leaving the consulting room. Doctors tend to want to take action but sometimes it is best to decide to do nothing — 'masterly inactivity'.

Qualifications to Pendleton et al's suggestions
• There is rarely enough time to perform the 'ideal' consultation. • Problems are not presented all at once or in order of importance. • The more problems that are dealt with, the less likely they are to be dealt with well. • Many symptoms may suggest an unconnected cause, e.g. depression. • Patients may 'test the water' with a minor symptom before trusting the doctor with the main problem. • The most important information is often given just as the patient is leaving. • 'Masterly inactivity' may be an appropriate treatment.

A more recent analysis of the consultation has been provided by Roger Neighbour (1987) in his book *The Inner Consultation*. He presents a model of consulting as a progression towards five successive 'checkpoints'.

These are described as:

- Connecting
- Summarising
- Handing-over
- Safety-netting
- Housekeeping

'Connecting' means being able to see the problem as the patient does. 'Summarising' is telling the patient the impression you have so far formed of their needs. 'Handing-over' is telling the patient how you see the situation and how you suggest proceeding from this point on. Handing-over would always include the opportunity for the patient to comment on your assessment and ask further questions. 'Safety-netting' means anticipating what might happen next to the patient, for example, explaining what effect you would expect some treatment to have and what you would plan to do next if this was not the case. 'Housekeeping' refers to dealing with the feelings left by one consultation before moving on to the next.

Communication style in the consultation

Sociologists have suggested that the styles adopted by doctors and patients may be those thought most likely to satisfy their own needs. Styles might be adopted to maximise reward, the doctor wanting to feel useful and the patient wanting to feel better. Past experience and social class are thought to be major influences on communication style. For those who have received a medical training, the effect of exposure to medical teachers is another powerful influence and it is salutary to remember that this sort of modelling may have both positive and negative effects.

There are protagonists for both 'authoritarian' and 'sharing' communication styles adopted by doctors. Authoritarian doctors argue that by exerting power and expecting obedience from patients they take responsibility for the medical condition. Patients, in losing freedom, also shed the anxiety that goes with responsibility of trying to make themselves feel better. The energy saved can then be directed towards getting better by cooperating with a trusted expert.

Advocates of the sharing style suggest that today's patients expect to be more autonomous and to be more involved in making decisions. They are better able to do this because education and increased media coverage on medical matters mean that they are better informed. There are still many chronic physical and psychiatric illnesses that are not curable. In these cases particularly, the patient's cooperation and involvement in management will help the doctor to control symptoms and maximise function. Patients with chronic disease often know more about their condition than their doctor. Modern medical treatment has become extremely expensive and patients, who are also tax payers, might wish to be involved in decisions about allocation of resources. There is also medico-legal pressure towards the sharing style as it is thought that shared decision making is less likely to end in litigation. A sharing style is beneficial, especially when negotiating health education and prevention issues with patients.

Clinical research using patient satisfaction as a measure of communication style when giving advice and treatment in general practice suggests that simple physical illness responding to the traditional biomedical approach of diagnosis and treatment is best suited to a directing style. For the increasing number of consultations for patients with illnesses that have a large psychosocial component the traditional biomedical model manages poorly, and the benefit of a directing style disappears (Savage & Armstrong 1990).

Could it be that after decades of exposure to bossy doctors patients expect such behaviour? Might there be a gain for patients in handing responsibility for illness or problems to the doctor and might this behaviour make their doctor feel important? What communication styles do colleagues use and how effective are they? The trainee year should offer you the opportunity to explore and experiment with communication styles and to develop ways of becoming more effective at communicating.

Summary: the theory of the consultation

Different accounts of the theory of the consultation include:

- Balint (1957)
- Byrne & Long (1976)
- Pendleton et al (1984)
- Neighbour (1987).

Influences on communication in the consultation:

- the doctor and patient as people
- the doctor's view of her/himself
- past experience
- the perceived needs of doctor and patient
- maximising the chances of feeling useful and of being rewarded
- modelling on teachers
- repetitive nature of the consultation
- time constraints
- doctor's communication style.

Some specific examples of communication skills used in the consultation

The following section draws on the psychology of communication and applies it to the general practice consultation.

Active listening

Listening involves hearing and interpreting. Many steps are involved in these processes:

- Sound has to be received.
- It is then matched with previous knowledge of similar sounds to confirm it has been heard accurately.
- Comparison with existing knowledge of grammar will then allow a sequence of matched sounds to be accepted as a sentence.
- The identified language is analysed to discover its meaning. This is deduced from the choice and combination of words.
- The context of the sentence is examined and influences the understanding of what is said (about 75% of language is involved with transmitting context).
- Personal knowledge and beliefs are then incorporated to make a decision about whether to accept the utterance as personally valid.

Each of the many stages described influences understanding of what is said. While superficial understanding may allow simple problems to be dealt with, more complex problems require deeper analysis.

On being a better listener

Hear what is being said The first and perhaps most difficult step is to believe that what is being said is worth listening to. This is made easier if patients are thought of as equals with particular expertise relating to their own problem.

Try hard to listen with your *full* attention. Other thinking must be suspended. Don't go through your history-taking checklist or wonder what examination to do, just listen. Suspend judgement about the problem so that attention is focused on what is being said. Note-taking should be kept to a minimum and done as unobtrusively as possible as it is inevitable that this will interrupt your communication. Minimise interruptions from other practice team members, the telephone and extraneous noise.

Encourage the patient to tell you the problem This may not be difficult if the problem is an upper respiratory tract infection but for more complicated, concealed problems:

- *Be interested* in what is being said. Valuing the patient encourages them to disclose their problem.
- *Let the patient speak first.*
- *Affirm* what is being said: encouraging grunts and nods give confidence to the patient to continue.
- Be encouraging by *confirming* that what is being said is important or that it has been courageous or useful to have said it.
- Use *reflection*. This is a way of encouraging the patient to continue by picking up and repeating a phrase or idea they have just used.
- Don't be afraid of *silence*. Let the patient dictate the pace. Be patient: don't try to hurry the conversation by finishing sentences if the patient falters; this may make them feel inadequate and stop them telling you their real concerns.
- *Clarify* at intervals. Appropriate prompts can help to make clear what the patient is trying to put into words. Use the minimum input, however, to direct the patient's attention to the main problem and avoid the temptation to lead the patient towards your line of thought.
- *Summarise* the patient's account from time to time. This is a way of both checking that you have understood what the patient means to say and also demonstrating that you are listening and understanding.
- As the problem unfolds it may be helpful to show that you identify with the patient's experience.

Relating to the dilemma encourages the patient to reveal more personal information. Be careful though, it may not be helpful to the patient to start sharing your own experience or to seem to want them to counsel you.

It is not unusual for people to become upset and show their emotions in the doctor's surgery. It is not because people sneeze a lot that most GPs keep a box of tissues on their desk! Sometimes it seems that just closing the door of the consulting room is a trigger for tears. You may find that if you use the active listening approach outlined above even more of your patients will display their emotions. People are often apologetic when they become upset, but these reactions should be regarded as positive and therapeutic as long as you are able to deal with them in a constructive and sensitive way. As a first response a few moments silence is often helpful. You can then say something to *mirror* or *confront* their feelings, such as simply 'That must make you feel very upset'. This gives *permission* to patients to let go of pent-up emotion, and allows you to help them come to terms with their distress.

Listening to what is not said Sometimes what is left unsaid may be the vital issue. Hearing what is not said is a difficult skill but becomes easier as the relationship with the patient becomes established. A sore throat may be presented, but smudged make-up and downcast eyes tell of another problem altogether. The anxious daughter who attends for another course of antibiotics for her bronchitis but omits any discussion about her dying mother may need an opportunity to talk about the strain she is under.

Listening to what a question is saying Questions are also statements as they hint at the questioner's view on the subject. The patient who asks about a sickness certificate has a view of their own ability to return to work. It is worthwhile exploring rather than assuming the implication behind questions.

Listen to be therapeutic Attending to the patient gives them a sense of worth and tells them that you value what they are saying. This is more likely to make the patient feel that the problem has been properly addressed and therefore will make them more confident when embarking on the advice or treatment offered.

Admit when you are lost If you have lost the thread or run out of energy or concentration and can no longer listen, the patient may sense this and interpret it as indifference. It may be better to acknowledge the problem to the patient who can then choose whether to continue or return to see you at another time.

If you discover you have not been listening:

- Apologise and ask the patient to repeat what you missed.
- Summarise to check understanding.
- If the other thoughts won't go away you may have to deal with them first.
- You may be too tired to continue listening. As soon as possible have a short break, walk up and down the corridor or get a (non-alcoholic) drink.

Exercises to improve listening skills

- Practise different ways of behaving in the consultation. See if your new style improves communication.
- Discuss videotapes of your consultations with someone you trust.
- Check what you are thinking about as the consultation proceeds. You are probably not listening effectively if you are pondering a diagnosis, an investigation or what to say next.

Listening with your eyes (non-verbal cues)

If listening is an extremely complicated process it is further compounded by information gleaned from what is seen. What is seen is often more startling because it is not altered or censored by the brain to the extent that speech is. Ears and eyes gather information and one informs the other.

The doctor's first impression of the patient on entering the consulting room starts to focus the mind even before a conversation starts. The initial appraisal may involve relatively fixed cues such as:

- physique
- colour of skin
- face
- clothes
- make-up
- cleanliness
- hair style.

No matter how liberal we may like to think we are, we all have some positive or negative prejudices and visual clues often tend to trigger our preconceived notions. This may be very misleading and distort our assessment, so it is important to be aware of personal prejudice and to check impressions with the patient. Prejudice about obesity may suggest such diverse causes as gluttony or depression while personal knowledge of an individual can suggest a more accurate impression such as genetic influence, different cultural ideas of beauty (obesity is considered attractive by many Africans) or a diagnosis of Cushing's syndrome. An attractive face may make a doctor more receptive and friendly or inhibited and shy.

Voice quality and accent are strong generators of prejudice, especially for those educated in the United Kingdom where accents can be badges of class and personal values. Clothes and hair style send out strong signals about how individuals would like others to classify them: punks and Rastafarians are two examples. Self-neglect may signal poverty, drug abuse, low intelligence or depression but may be related to poor housing, marital disharmony or numerous other causes.

Previous knowledge of the patient allows comparison of more dynamic non-verbal cues:

- body posture
- movements
- gestures
- facial expression
- eye movements
- speech, especially tone, rate and fluency.

Body posture can be an indicator of mood. The way the patient walks may indicate confidence, dignity, fear or anxiety. The patient may sit on the edge of the chair with a rigid back indicating tension or may sit comfortably relaxed against the back of the chair. Leaning forward may indicate urgency or anger while leaning back with arms and legs crossed may indicate reluctance to talk.

Body movements such as nodding, shaking the head or shrugging the shoulders have well-recognised meanings. Be aware, however, of possible cultural differences in the use of body movements; for example, some people from Southern Asia may affirm by shaking the head in a way that signals denial to most Europeans. Use of gestures may illustrate a description or indicate the severity of a symptom, while wringing of hands may indicate anxiety. Sloping the head to one side or looking 'hangdog' while speaking may indicate resignation that nothing can be done.

Eye contact is a powerful way of influencing communication. Sympathetic eye contact can encourage the patient to speak, especially when combined with appropriate pauses and encouraging body language. It shows that the doctor is paying attention and values the patient. Be aware of prolonged eye contact, which may be a sign of heightened emotions such as anger or helplessness. Staring can be threatening and may make the patient want to leave the consultation. By way of contrast, avoidance of eye contact may indicate guilt, for example, failure to comply with prescribed treatment. It may also suggest fear, for example, of a serious diagnosis such as cancer. Depression may also reduce eye contact. A darting gaze may indicate anxiety.

Touch

Touch can have a powerful effect in the consultation. A hand on the shoulder or on the patient's hand can often reinforce care or concern felt by the doctor and convey reassurance to the patient. Touch can be especially helpful when communicating with the elderly, children or adults who may be lonely or isolated. It may be a better method of communication than words, for example, after tragic news has been broken. The use of touch is a very personal thing and may not be comfortable for all of us. You must decide how you feel about it and gauge each patient as an individual.

Giving effective information and advice

Good communication requires skills in both receiving and giving information. Just stating facts or advice does not guarantee that they will be understood or retained.

The most common complaint made by patients is that their doctor failed to give them enough information. Inadequate time for communication, lack of sensitivity to the patient's needs and failure to understand their concerns are other sources of complaint. The type of language we use is vital to patient understanding and satisfaction. We must be able to vary this according to factors such as the patient's age, education, understanding of English, social background and culture.

Medical jargon confuses patients. Doctors use jargon for many reasons:

- to streamline conversation
- to save time
- to appear knowledgeable and powerful
- to boost self-confidence
- to hide ignorance
- to confuse or silence the patient.

Patients will often fail to challenge the use of medical jargon. They may feel flattered that the doctor is treating them as well-informed or they may not wish to appear ignorant.

Information may not be communicated effectively because patients possess different medical knowledge from doctors. The patient's idea of the site or function of internal organs may be very different from the doctor's perception.

Patients' experience of illness may also differ from the doctor's:

An African mother of a 3-month-old baby burst into tears when told her son had conjunctivitis; discharge from the eyes in her country means blindness from trachoma.

Patients do frequently misunderstand their doctor's instructions and advice. For example, physiotherapists often see patients with back problems sleeping on boards on top of their mattresses when the doctors are certain they advised putting the board under the mattress. Misinterpretation of advice about medication and diet is commonplace, for example, about when to take medication in relation to meal times.

About half of the advice given in a consultation is not remembered for any length of time. For this reason it is important to give simple, specific advice that is:

- understandable
- emphasised
- organised into categories
- relevant to the patient's specific anxieties and concerns.

Simple written instructions or advice can reinforce what is said. Clearly written leaflets about management of conditions are useful and should be provided when possible in the patient's first language.

Giving patients their medical records can enhance communication. Obstetric patients who look after their own records have demonstrated that not only are they more efficient at keeping them than the hospital medical records department but also their reading of them stimulates questioning and allows better understanding of the purpose of antenatal care. The improved communication has resulted in better attendance at the antenatal clinic and lower perinatal mortality in some practices.

When giving information to patients:

- Use language tailored to each patient's needs.
- Be concrete and specific. The advice 'walk for at least one mile a day' is more likely to be followed than general advice, such as 'take more exercise'.
- Focus on the 'here and now'. What is happening at the present moment and how to progress in the future are of most importance.
- Resist giving advice early on. This allows the patient to remain in control so strategies can be developed jointly if appropriate. Giving advice allows the patient only two options, to accept with the risk of feeling passive or to decline with the risk of feeling isolated and unsupported.
- Don't give advice if it is not wanted. It may be that the problem is still being explored or deciphered, and emotions may block information offered.
- Don't give more information and advice than the patient can cope with. It has been suggested that three pieces of information is the maximum that patients are likely to retain when they leave the consultation.
- Repeat important messages and ask patients to repeat them to you in order to check understanding.
- Reinforce important messages by writing them down for the patient to take away.

Patients who are satisfied with communication in the consultation are more likely to be compliant with treatment. In other words, your medical education is wasted unless you are a good communicator. Also, you are the most unreliable judge of your communication skills; so, out with the video camera or tape recorder, find a sympathetic friend and compare communication skills!

Summary: communication skills

Listening

- Give full attention and value what is being said.
- Encourage the patient using:
  - affirmation
  - confirmation
  - reflection
  - silence
  - clarification
  - summarising
  - mirroring
  - confronting
  - permitting.

Seeing

- Watch for non-verbal clues:
  - appearance
  - posture
  - body movement
  - speech.
- Think about eye contact.

Touching

- Use touch when it is appropriate and comfortable.

Information giving

- Tailor your language.
- Be concrete and specific.
- Don't give advice too early or too much.
- Repeat important messages.
- Reinforce advice with written material.

BREAKING NEWS

By giving the result of an investigation, informing about the outcome of an intervention or a decision, doctors are breaking news all the time almost without thinking about it. News is given by doctors or other staff to patients face to face, by telephone or by letter.

News, while sometimes representing the end of the diagnostic process for the doctor, may be the start of the patient's problems. Take the result of a pregnancy test for example. A positive test may be disastrous for an unmarried teenager who has just broken up with her boyfriend while a negative result would be equally disastrous for a woman who has been trying to conceive for many months in a relationship which depends on fertility for its continuation.

- Give news and other information simply and clearly. The patient who is waiting for news will be in a heightened emotional state that may hamper understanding.
- News should be given calmly and with care.
- Give the patient time to consider the news.
- Check out understanding of what has been said.

Often the way news is misunderstood gives an early clue as to the fears of the patient about what might be wrong.

- It is important to discuss the implications and the emotions that the news generates.

- Watch body language; this may give the first clue as to the meaning of the news.
- Encouragement and support may be important. If the news has caused confusion, offer another consultation in a few days when the patient has had time to consider.
- Some news, for example, about a condition such as sickle cell disease, may be followed up by use of explanatory leaflets. Leaflets, used on their own, help patients remember about 10% of the information. When given with a general explanation retention increases to 30% but with personally constructed advice and a leaflet information retained can be as much as 70%.

Breaking bad news

Tragic news, such as the discovery of a cancer, may produce a sequence of emotions over a period of time similar to that which accompanies bereavement. The initial shock and denial may give way to anger. The patient may seek someone to blame for the tragedy and depression and guilt may follow.

Patients may use selective hearing to filter out or reinterpret what is unacceptable to them. It may be helpful to check what the bad news means to the patient who may have drawn erroneous conclusions. Patients who believe they have little control over their lives fare better with more general explanations while those who feel able to exert control over external events prefer more detailed explanation.

Much can be done by personal involvement that includes support and a positive approach to the management of the patient's problem. This longer-term support may require the agreement of some boundaries in order to manage time and the patient's expectations of the doctor.

The balance between the ideal care of the patient and the right of the doctor to limit availability and involvement is sometimes hard to achieve. Such compromises are best made when problems and concerns are shared.

TALKING TO ANGRY PATIENTS

The angry patient is in an emotionally charged state. Doctors will react in different ways but the preferred response is to adopt as neutral a position as possible. Try to remain calm and sympathetic showing understanding and concern. This allows careful listening to extract the source of the anger from emotionally charged rhetoric. A neutral and attentive doctor is less likely to fuel the anger further. An unaggressive body posture, facing the patient and meeting the increased eye contact with a concentrated gaze is probably best.

In most situations it is reasonable to assume that 'the customer is always right' at least initially until the source of anger is discovered. Possible problems include:

- A phrase may have been misheard or a misunderstanding arisen, in which case gentle and sensitive explanation may solve the problem.
- A genuine mistake may have been made; its admission may defuse the situation.
- The patient's expectations of the profession or services offered may be unreasonable, in which case gentle but firm statement of the professional boundaries may not stem the anger but may allow the patient to reflect once the anger subsides.
- The patient may be psychiatrically disturbed, in which case personal safety of the patient and doctor must be the priority.
- Patients may be angry with other doctors or members of staff so the doctor may have to explain or mediate.

It is important to have (and show when appropriate) self-belief, and to be confident within the limitations of the general practitioner's professional role.

When apologising, it is important to distinguish between sorrow and guilt over what has happened. Feeling guilty may be inappropriate and lead the patient to think that the doctor has been negligent. Doctors are also allowed to show their feelings, and this includes anger, but matching anger with anger closes down communication and polarises views so that it is hard to continue to be available and useful to that patient.

Inflated expectations of medicine sometimes fanned by ambitious claims in the press are producing more angry patients (a 50% increase in complaints and litigation in 1990). The doctor-patient relationship may be weakened by a less personal service as sub-specialisation develops in response to demands for greater efficiency.

TALKING TO PATIENTS ON THE TELEPHONE

This is an important skill, not least because it is the usual way patients communicate with their doctor when the surgery is closed. Out-of-hours telephone conversations usually deal with acute problems biased towards children and the elderly.

When dealing with visit requests the golden rule is never to refuse to visit. Many complaints and much litigation occur as a result of such refusal. A visit when tired or exhausted may save what can be years of guilt about a missed diagnosis, and the stress resulting from defending a complaint or preparing for a court appearance. If the mental attitude is adopted from the moment you pick up the phone that 'of course I will visit if you want' this places responsibility on the patient, whose task changes from persuading the doctor to visit to deciding with the doctor's help if the condition is serious enough to warrant a visit to the home. Inappropriate calls may be reduced by ensuring that the purpose and arrangements for out-of-hours cover are known and understood by patients. This can be outlined in the practice leaflet and explained to all newly registering patients.

Understandably, doctors don't like being disturbed and may protect themselves by being dismissive, implying that the condition phoned about is trivial or transmitting in other ways their frustration at being called. Patients are usually anxious and think they are unwell when they phone; they need their problem to be discussed, the possibilities explored and a prognosis and strategies for management offered.

Doctors are either optimists or pessimists. Optimists expect that symptoms will usually be explained by a common self-limiting condition while pessimists feel it necessary to exclude serious illness. The former must guard against unreasonable reassurance or missed diagnoses, and the latter against frustration with the patient when serious illness is excluded. Research has shown that more than half of patients managed by telephone advice subsequently attended surgery for the same problem with no detriment to their health.

Telephone conversations tend to be more structured, more to do with the doctor's agenda and contain more direct questions to exclude potentially serious conditions. Much useful information can be missed by failing to ask about past outcome of similar symptoms and of the personal meaning of the present problem. Genuine calmness and sympathy for the dilemma pass down telephone lines remarkably easily and are very therapeutic. Confidence in your own assessment of the problem coupled with a clear simple explanation will further help.

If you have difficulty being assertive on the telephone try standing up when you speak as this helps you to talk with more authority.

A relative may phone on the patient's behalf; always ask if it is possible to speak to the patient as their assessment may differ and it may be the relative who needs the advice, reassurance or 'treatment'.

Telephone interruptions during consultations can be a particular irritation. It is important to take the patient's and the telephonist's difficulties into account when developing a strategy. If it takes half an hour to get through to the surgery the patient will not be pleased at being asked to call back later and the telephonist will not be pleased at receiving the subsequent abuse about difficulty getting through on the phone. Some consultations can't be interrupted and it is appropriate to tell the telephonist this, but being permanently unobtainable is not reasonable. Practice routines that delegate giving test results over the phone make telephone use more efficient. Agreed protocols to deal with the clinical consequences of an abnormal result lessen the thinking burden of an interruption.

Some doctors have developed a 'telephone surgery', time set aside when patients know that telephone queries can be dealt with. Again, these can be detailed in the practice leaflet.

Finally, it is wise to record telephone conversations with patients in their notes with the date and time. Some practices also log all incoming telephone calls and keep records for reference or for medico-legal purposes.

COMMUNICATION OUTSIDE THE CONSULTATION

A general practitioner has to develop communication skills to be a:

- businessman
- employer
- motivator
- disciplinarian
- negotiator
- collaborator
- liaison officer
- politician
- innovator.

One study identified 97 different people that general practitioners communicate with about their patients!

Communicating with your trainer

Most trainees get on well with their trainer but a minority have problems. The change from the hierarchical hospital relationship will be helped by defining the trainee's responsibilities and boundaries as early as possible in the general practice attachment. Working through a model trainee contract such as that produced by the BMA is a useful exercise because it draws attention to obligations and potential problem areas. It also gives trainee and trainer a chance to start negotiating with each other. As the attachment progresses unforeseen situations will occur and good communications are vital to a working relationship that may explore solutions by renegotiating prior agreements.

On being assertive

This section describes principles that apply to effective communication — whether it be with trainers, partners, patients or others. Some trainees find it difficult to defend their point of view. Emotional blocks such as anger may obstruct reasoning or insight. While it is not desirable to bully or be stubborn, being assertive is essential for effective communication.

Trainees must feel responsible for, and in control of, their actions so that they can recognise what they want and ask openly and directly for it. Not feeling in complete control may mean:

- not defending or valuing oneself enough to argue one's point of view
- being angry or upset
- being aggressive
- aiming to get one's own way and disregarding the other person's feelings
- being passive and avoiding decisions with the result of feeling helpless or unfairly treated
- being manipulative.

Openness and honesty at work and in personal relationships with staff engender trust and respect so that a request is more likely to be acknowledged and considered.

The trainer has needs and rights too and these must also be respected. Negotiation and compromise are skills needed to make both parties feel justly treated. It is not helpful to see situations as 'win or lose'.

Essentials of assertiveness

- Have enough composure to know what you want.
- Be open and honest.
- Acknowledge that your trainer has needs and rights too.
- Negotiation and compromise are important skills.

Assertiveness is important to maintain self-esteem and to be effective. In order to have the best chance of success in a negotiation it is important to pick the right time for discussion:

- There must be enough time.
- The time must be protected from outside interruptions or other pressures.
- Both parties must be receptive.

Setting the scene

- Only talk about a problem when you are ready, 'I am happy to talk about this but not now', and fix a time when you are prepared and unlikely to be interrupted.
- Conduct your conversation sitting. If your trainer is standing then ask him or her to sit too. If you both stand you risk a more confrontational exchange. There is a place for confrontation occasionally but it is advisable to keep the emotional temperature as low as possible.
- Sit with your bottom at the back of the chair, keeping your back straight, and breathe slowly and deeply. Have your legs and arms unfolded. Use direct eye contact.

Here is a checklist to use before entering a negotiation:

1. Am I in control of myself?
- too tired?
- angry or depressed?
- anxious or stressed?
- feel beaten before I start?

2. What is the real problem?
- Do I understand the problem?
- What am I still unclear about?
- What could confuse or put the argument off course?
- Do we both agree this is the real problem?

3. How is my trainer feeling?
- What can be reasonably expected of my trainer?
- What might be of concern to my trainer?
- Are there any other problems I don't know about?
- Is my trainer angry or upset?

4. How can we both win?
- What can we negotiate about to get close to what we both want?

5. Act early to avoid a build-up of issues.
- What is the key issue? A single action such as a change in the on-call rota may have many subsequent effects. The main issue may then become obscured.

6. Speak simply and honestly.
- Use 'I' statements —'I would like ... want ... think ... feel.' 'It is important to me that you take me seriously.'

7. Be sure that you are being heard.
- If not, say 'I feel it is important you listen to me'. 'It is important to me that you take me seriously.'

8. Are you both talking about the same thing?
- If not and there are several issues to talk about, agree to choose one to work on.

9. Describe your feelings.
- Tell the other person how you are feeling as the conversation progresses.

10. Don't bale out under pressure.
- Tension in the conversation may be necessary so:
    — Don't apologise inappropriately or use other rescuing tactics.
    — If tension makes you feel uncomfortable, practice living with it.

11. Be positive.
- Make choices and feel in control.
- Avoid statements that belittle each other. If you are receiving put-down statements it may be because the other person can only feel comfortable and in control if you are not!

12. Explore your trainer's point of view.
- This avoids focusing on the weakness of your own arguments.

13. You don't have to state your position if you don't want to.
- Don't be drawn to say something you don't want to, it's permissible to decide not to comment on some things.

14. Watch for 'dirty tricks'.
- Your trainer may try to pull rank by talking in generalities, for example, 'none of the other trainees has had this problem'. Counteract this by requesting you both use 'I' statements and asking for *your* problems to be the focus of attention.
- Your trainer may try to blame your psychology or personality as the cause of the problem that can be 'treated' by him. This can be countered by being extra simple and straight but by leaving out the 'I feel' to concentrate on the material issues rather than your psyche.
- Don't be bullied or hurried; if you don't understand, say so.

15. You don't have to win to win.
- Be prepared to leave the discussion having presented yourself well but not having got what you wanted. You will have gained better understanding of yourself, your trainer and the pressures both of you are under. In this way you retain your dignity and the knowledge gained makes you a more formidable force to deal with in the future. Some situations may provide valuable learning outcomes despite loss of the argument.

More tips on negotiation

- If you disagree, listen harder and you will learn more about your trainer's point of view.
- Monitor your feelings. You can double check by noting your pulse, respiratory rate, the tension in the muscles at the back of your neck and watching what your hands are doing.
- If you start to get upset, listen harder because it probably means a weakness in your argument has been exposed.
- Words can generate strong emotions. The purpose of emotion is to make people act effectively but it can have the opposite action in an argument. Watch out for words that upset people. Tone down the emotional content of what is said in an argument, try to think in neutral words and don't polarise. Examination of the emotional words being used may give new insight into the factual and moral strands of the argument.

- Prejudice arises from ignoring evidence that does not support one's point of view. Questioning assumptions that support arguments may lead to a more rational and balanced view.
- Be aware that habitual thoughts have not closed your mind to new ideas.
- What matters is what is heard, not what is said; don't be afraid to check your trainer's understanding of what has been said — their experience may be different from your own.
- Avoid thinking ahead. You think faster than your trainer can talk, so slow down and stay with the conversation in order not to get confused.
- Ensure that the conversation is always on an adult level. If your trainer starts talking like a parent tell them how it makes you feel.

Communication and the practice team

Many practice 'teams' may exist in name only, functioning more like associations or hierarchies of health professionals. There may also be varying views about who should be the 'team captain' or manager if one is needed. Real teamwork requires that the team members:

- value each other
- appreciate each others' skills
- understand each others' different priorities, responsibilities and background
- want to work together
- are prepared to support each other
- have a common sense of purpose or common goals
- are prepared to give time to make the team work.

Different relationships within the team can create tension. For example, the practice may employ a nurse who sees her loyalties in a different way from the District Health Authority employed nurse working in the same practice. Being employed by the practice may constrain or enable the directly employed nurse, depending on personality and professional aims, while the district nurse may feel that a remote administration does not understand fully the problems of delivering community nursing care or that the doctors do not understand the nursing role in the community.

Receptionists are employed by the practice and are answerable to the doctors but they want to provide a good service for the patients and often feel frustrated by divided loyalties when, for example, there are more requests for appointments than available spaces.

It is important to appreciate the expertise of team members. The community nurse may be the expert in caring for a dying patient while the receptionist's encyclopedic knowledge of the practice clientele is invaluable.

A successful team needs good management. There needs to be:

- good communication between members

- agreed lines of delegation
- agreed areas of responsibility
- agreed procedures to follow when things go wrong.

In order to achieve these aims, time needs to be reserved in the busy working week for all team members to meet regularly. The meetings need a clear agenda to avoid the feeling of wasting valuable time when 'work' could be done. Team members need to be good listeners, as already described in this chapter.

The trainee may either be welcomed into the team or be kept as an outsider. It is vital to be able to work with practice staff but not to be put upon by them. Being friendly but also assertive should enable the best chance of achieving a satisfactory relationship with the practice team.

Letters to hospital consultants

Most GPs take considerable care in writing thorough referral letters about their patients and yet there is evidence to show that the letters are rarely carefully read by consultants and much is said of their deficiencies. At worst, they become a labour-intensive method of securing an outpatient appointment, at best they are an effective patient-centred method of communication and mutual education between doctors. They are the most common method of communication between general practitioners and consultants, and the correspondence that follows can provide an opportunity for GPs to keep up-to-date with specialty learning and be a useful addition to the patient's records.

The most important functions of the referral letter are to:

- state the reason for making the referral
- ask questions
- request an investigation
- define the limits of intervention by a consultant
- impart information that might not be known
- indicate when it is possible to resume care of the patient in the community
- clarify what community services and support are currently available.

It is important that the letter is legible, that the patient understands the procedure for making the outpatient appointment (or when to expect an appointment to be sent), and that they know when to ask if nothing is heard from the hospital or if the appointment is too far in the future.

It is reasonable to complain (in a constructive way) if discharge letters are not received or are unduly delayed. 'We don't have any secretaries' may reflect the consultant's views of the importance of communicating with GPs rather than his ability to organise his department.

Spend some time thinking about the way you write referral letters and ask your trainer to read some of them and feed back comments to you. It is also worthwhile to look back in patients' notes at letters written by other doctors and compare the different styles used.

CONCLUSION

This chapter has aimed to stress the central importance of effective and sympathetic communication in general practice, both within and outside the special setting of the consultation. The way we communicate is influenced by our personality and experience and varies with circumstances. Your basic skills can, however, be built on and refined by thinking about the theory of communication, learning some simple rules, and examining your current practice. Advice has been given on dealing with some of the situations which make up the work of the GP. Although much of what has been said could equally apply to any situation where one is dealing with people, it is the close relationships which we develop, often over many years, with patients, colleagues and staff which make this topic so vital to general practitioners.

There is no single 'right' way to communicate or to consult. It is hoped, however, that the ideas contained within this chapter will provide some signposts to stimulate your thinking and help you to develop your own unique and personal style of communication.

REFERENCES

Balint M 1957 The doctor, his patient and the illness, Tunbridge Wells. Pitman Medical, Tunbridge Wells
Byrne P, Long B 1976 Doctors talking to patients. HMSO, London
Neighbour R 1987 The inner consultation. MTP Press, Lancaster
Pendleton D, Schofield T, Tate P, Havelock P 1984 The consultation: an approach to learning and teaching. Oxford University Press, Oxford
Savage R, Armstrong D 1990 Effect of a general practitioner's style on patients' satisfaction: a controlled study. British Medical Journal 301: 968–970
Stott N C H, Davies R H 1979 The exceptional potential in each primary care consultation. Journal of the Royal College of General Practitioners 29: 201–205
Zborowski M 1952 Cultural components in response to pain. Journal of Social Issues 8: 16–30

FURTHER READING

THE ROLE OF THE DOCTOR

Berger J, Mohr P 1967 A fortunate man. Penguin, London
Brody H 1987 Stories of sickness. Yale University Press, New Haven, USA
Tudor-Hart J 1988 A new kind of doctor. Merlin, London

LAY EXPERIENCE OF MEDICINE

Helman C G 1978 Feed a cold and starve a fever: folk models of infection in an English suburban community and their relation to medical treatment. Culture, Medicine and Psychiatry 2 (2): 107–137
Tuckett D, Boulton M, Olson C, Williams A 1985 Meetings between experts: an approach to sharing ideas in medical consultations. Tavistock, London

THE CONSULTATION

Katon W, Kleinman A 1980 Doctor-patient negotiation and other social science strategies in patient care. In: Eisenberg L, Kleinman A (eds) The relevance of social science for medicine. Reidel, Dorbrecht

PSYCHOLOGY OF COMMUNICATION

Miller G A 1968 The psychology of communication: seven essays. Penguin, Harmondsworth

5. Disease prevention and health promotion in practice

Margaret Lloyd

INTRODUCTION

The diagnosis and management of disease are often seen as being more interesting and challenging than preventing disease and promoting health. However, an increasing proportion of those involved in health care share the frustration of the physician in Zola's parable of the river of disease. He paints a picture in words of a river in which people are being swept downstream, many drowning. A doctor stands on the bank, applying artificial respiration to a man he has just pulled from the flood. He wishes that he had time to prevent them falling in upstream, or even to throw them a life-raft or ring, which at least some of them could take advantage of.

This chapter will look at the scope in general practice for preventing disease and promoting health, the underlying principles involved and how best we can accept the challenge. This is an enormous field to cover in one chapter and it cannot be a comprehensive account of all preventive activities carried out in general practice. The aim is to help the trainee to think critically about what is done in the name of disease prevention and health promotion.

The first section will deal with basic definitions, the scope for prevention, the roles of government and the primary health care team, and the theoretical concepts underlying screening and health education activities. The second section will cover the more practical aspects of disease prevention and health promotion in general practice.

PRINCIPLES OF DISEASE PREVENTION AND HEALTH PROMOTION

Defining the terms

First of all, what is meant by the terms disease prevention and health promotion? Within the context of general practice the preventive activities which most readily come to mind include immunisation, cervical screening and advising patients about stopping smoking. These activities aim to prevent disease or ill-health. But health is not merely the absence of disease; it also has a positive component, described in the WHO definition as 'a state of complete physical, mental and social well being'. This definition has been criticised as being too idealistic but it does stress the positive side of health. Our role is not only to prevent disease but to help patients to achieve, as far as possible, this state of wellbeing.

> **DISCUSSION POINT**
>
> **Definitions**
>
> Read (or re-read) Chapter • and think about the meaning of the following terms:
> — ill-health
> — positive health
> — prevention
> — health promotion.

Health promotion has been defined as 'the efforts to enhance positive health and prevent ill-health through the overlapping spheres of health education, prevention and health protection' (Downie et al 1990; Fig. 5.1).

Health promotion emphasises the dual role of preventing ill-health and promoting positive health; Figure 5.1 illustrates the three overlapping approaches. The primary health care team are predominantly involved in prevention and health education. Health protection activities lie more in the public health domain.

Prevention

Prevention is about reducing the risk of a disease process, illness, injury or disability. It includes preventive services, e.g. immunisation and screening, preventive health education, e.g. advice about sensible drinking, and preventive health protection., e.g. taxing tobacco and fluoridating water (Fig. 5.1). Preventive activities are often classified as primary, secondary or tertiary prevention. These reflect the stages in the natural history of the disease at which the intervention is made.

Primary prevention includes all activities which remove the cause of disease or decrease the susceptibility of the individual to the causative agent. Many primary preventive activities should be part of the national strategy. In general practice, examples of primary prevention include:

- health education, e.g. advice about smoking
- immunisation.

Secondary prevention is the detection and treatment of disease before symptoms or disordered function develops., i.e. before irreversible damage occurs. Examples include:

- cervical screening
- screening for hypertension.

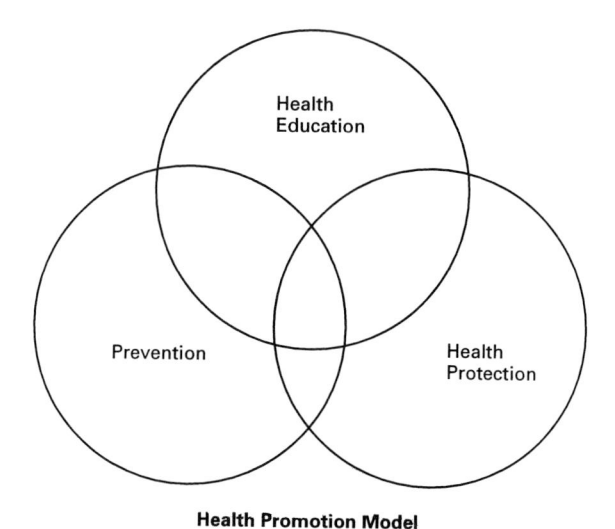

Fig. 5.1 A health promotion model. (After Downie et al 1990.)

Tertiary prevention is the monitoring and management of established disease in order to prevent disability or handicap. An example is:

- monitoring of patients with diabetes in order to detect and treat early complications.

This classification has been criticised by Tannahill (Downie et al 1990) on the grounds that it focuses on disease and includes treatment and that there is no standard definition of the terms primary, secondary and tertiary. For example, the term secondary prevention is sometimes used to describe interventions which aim to prevent recurrence of an illness, e.g. the use of aspirin and beta blockers after myocardial infarction. All classifications draw boundaries which at times seem artificial but they are useful as long as the reservations are borne in mind, and the classification of prevention is no exception to this.

Health education

Health education aims to diminish ill-health and enhance positive health by influencing people's beliefs, attitudes and behaviour. A central theme is helping (or empowering) individuals to build on their assets and to make appropriate choices for healthy living. This will be discussed in greater detail later in this chapter.

Health protection

Health protection activities are usually public health measures and include legal and fiscal controls and other regulations laid down by government.

These measures increase the chance of people living in a healthy environment and should help to make healthy choices easier choices.

The Peckham Experiment

The importance of linking disease prevention and health promotion was recognised in the 1920s when George Williamson and Innes Pearce set up the pioneer health centre at Peckham. This was a combined health centre and club for local families. The founders wanted to both study and cultivate health. The essential features of what has come to be known as the Peckham Experiment are as follows:

1. Health was considered to be much more than the absence of disease and as such deserved to be studied as a distinct entity.
2. There was a holistic approach to health which included the provision of a healthy environment and the promotion of social interaction between people.
3. There was an emphasis on the family unit. The whole family was encouraged to take part in social activities. They were offered regular health checks and the results were explained to the whole family at the family consultation.
4. The importance of non-directional self help was emphasised. People were encouraged to do things on their own initiative. There was open discussion between the members and the staff of the centre who worked together in an equal partnership.

The Peckham Experiment — with its emphasis on promoting good health rather than just preventing ill-health, the importance of the family unit and encouraging self help — is as relevant today as it was in the 1920s.

DISCUSSION POINT

The Peckham Experiment

— How might you introduce some of the concepts of the Peckham Experiment into a general practice?

Summary

1. Prevention of disease and promotion of health are two sides of the same coin.
2. Preventive activities can be classified as primary prevention (removing the cause of disease), secondary (screening) or tertiary prevention (preventing disability from established disease).

Prevention strategies

The scope for prevention

Where should efforts to prevent ill-health be directed? One approach is to look at the major causes of mortality and morbidity in the population today. At the beginning of this century, 40% of all deaths were due to infectious diseases. Now these account for a very small proportion of total deaths. Cancer, ischaemic heart disease, cerebrovascular disease and accidents have become the major causes of premature death (i.e. death before the age of 64 years) and total mortality, as shown in Figure 5.2.

Many of the risk factors associated with cancer and cardiovascular disease have been identified and are potentially modifiable. But prevention is not only about prolonging life, it is also about reducing morbidity, enabling

Causes of premature death in England (15 – 64 years) 1988

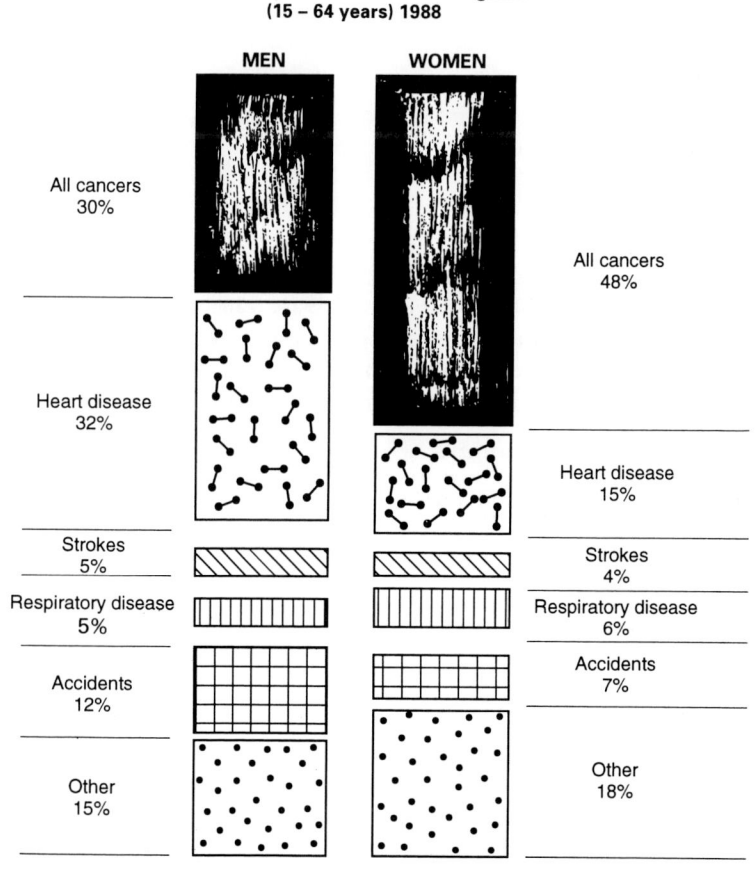

MEN — All cancers 30%; Heart disease 32%; Strokes 5%; Respiratory disease 5%; Accidents 12%; Other 15%.

WOMEN — All cancers 48%; Heart disease 15%; Strokes 4%; Respiratory disease 6%; Accidents 7%; Other 18%.

Fig. 5.2 Causes of premature death in England (15–64 years) in 1988. (Published by courtesy of the Health Education Authority.)

+---+
| **The scope for prevention** |
| |
| *Major causes of mortality*   *Major causes of morbidity* |
| • Coronary heart disease   • Mental illness |
| • Stroke   • Diabetes |
| • Cancer   • Asthma |
| • Accidents |
| |
| *Life-style risk factors contributing to mortality and morbidity* |
| • Smoking |
| • Diet |
| • Alcohol consumption |
| • Exercise |
| • Sexual behaviour |
+---+

people to lead fulfilling lives for as long as possible. Some key areas for prevention are listed above.

The Health of the Nation

In 1992 the Department of Health published a white paper *The Health of the Nation* (Secretary of State for Health 1992). This set out a strategy for improving the health of the population of England by identifying key areas for action, setting targets for reducing incidence in each area and suggesting strategies for achieving them by the year 2000 or 2010.

The key areas for action are:

- Coronary heart disease and stroke
- Cancers
- Mental illness
- HIV/AIDS and sexual health
- Accidents.

How are these targets to be achieved? A multi-pronged approach will be required, involving the following:

- the development of *public policies* (by government, industry, etc.) which take into account the health dimension;
- the development of *healthy surroundings* — in the home, in schools, at work, etc.;
- the adoption of *healthy life styles* by individuals;
- the delivery of high quality *health services*.

The importance of socioeconomic factors

The *Health of the Nation* document has been criticised for neglecting the relationship between health and socioeconomic factors. The persistent health gap between the social classes is a continuing cause for concern. In 1981 the standardised mortality ratio (SMR), which expresses age-adjusted death rates as a percentage of the average (which equals 100), was 66 for men in social class I and 129 for men in social classes IV and V. A similar gap is seen in infant mortality rates. In 1984 the rate in social class I was 8 per 1000 live births and in social class V it was 12 per 1000 live births. Children in the lower social classes are more likely to be born and brought up in conditions of poor housing, low income and poor nutrition, with unsupported mothers who are often smokers and stressed. Children who are socially and economically disadvantaged are more likely to have a low birth weight, which is strongly associated with neonatal death; they are more likely to develop respiratory illnesses; they are prone to accidents and are more likely to have behavioural problems and developmental delay. Improving social conditions and providing adequate financial and other support for disadvantaged families is the most effective way of preventing ill-health. Over the past 30 years the gap between the social classes has not only continued but has actually widened. Why should this be so?

The issue is a complex one but there is evidence that the gap is related to differences in income, housing conditions, employment and life style. This provides a challenge not only to the Government, but also to the primary health care team.

The role of the Government

Government policies and national strategies play a fundamental role in prevention. During the last century mortality from tuberculosis was falling long before the tubercle bacillus was identified and chemotherapy was developed, largely because of the improvement in nutrition and living conditions. Today, an increase in taxation on alcohol and tobacco would have a major effect on deaths from cardiovascular disease, cancer and accidents.

Strategies aimed at preventing ill-health should operate on at least four levels. For example, an effective programme to reduce alcohol-related problems and deaths might involve:

- *Government and national strategies*
  — Increased taxation on alcohol
  — Advertising restrictions
  — Changes in the law concerning drinking and driving.
- *District strategies*
  — Local health education programme about sensible drinking in schools and workplaces.

- *Practice strategies*
  — Increased efforts to identify and help individuals who are drinking at hazardous levels.
- *Individual strategies*
  — Each individual to review their alcohol consumption and to decide (with help if necessary) if they need to modify it.

The role of the primary health care team

The primary health care team has a unique role to play in the prevention of disease and the promotion of health. In the past, the role of the GP was seen in terms of responding to individuals who presented their problems to her/him. Diagnosis and management were the main activities of the general practitioner and prevention of disease was not a high priority. The move from this *reactive* form of care to *proactive* or *anticipatory* care gathered momentum in the 1970s. A Government report spoke of the new role of the general practitioner and included in the role:

The prevention of disease and *the maintenance of health* both physical and mental including the *detection of the earliest departure from normal* in the individuals and families of this population.

A major initiative by the Royal College of General Practitioners firmly established prevention and health promotion as a growth point in general practice. Their report stressed the importance of anticipatory care, i.e. anticipating people's problems and trying to prevent them from happening. Anticipatory care implies the union of prevention with care and cure. Care of the individual patient presenting with, for example, an upper respiratory tract infection, should include appropriate preventive activity, e.g. blood pressure screening.

In the 1990 Contract, prevention of disease became, for the first time, part of the general practitioner's terms of service.

A doctor shall render to his patients all necessary and appropriate personal medical services of the type usually provided by general practitioners including:

- Advice on general health
- Consultations and examinations to prevent disease.

In addition, the Government provided extra funds for health promotion in practices. Prevention of disease and promotion of health is now firmly established as an important part of the general practitioners' responsibility for which specific skills and training are necessary. This was recognised in the College publication *The Future General Practitioner* which was influential in setting the curriculum for vocational training and which included prevention-orientated objectives for the trainee.

The opportunities for disease prevention and health promotion in general practice are diverse and the most important ones are listed below.

Opportunities for prevention in general practice
Antenatal/children   • Cervical screening   • Antenatal care   • Blood pressure screening   • Smoking/alcohol in pregnancy   • Immunisation boosters   • Developmental screening   *Adolescence*   • Routine immunisations   • Contraception   • Accidents   • Safer sex   *Adults*   • Smoking   • Smoking   • Drugs   • Alcohol   • Rubella immunisation   • Diet   *Elderly*   • Exercise   • Screening for functional problems   • Contraception   • Safer sex   • Tetanus immunisation   • Breast screening   • Influenza immunisation

The general practitioner's responsibility is to care for both the individual patient are the whole practice population. Prevention strategies should be aimed at both the individual, particularly those at high risk, and the practice population.

High-risk and population strategies

There are two possible strategies for disease prevention and health promotion (Fig. 5.3). The *population* strategy aims to reduce the risk of the whole population, usually by public health measures. The *high-risk* strategy focuses on the individual who is considered to be at high risk.

The rationale behind the population strategy is that the bulk of the morbidity and mortality of a disease in a population is contributed by those who have a moderate degree of risk. For example, the British Regional Heart Study found that 60% of middle-aged British men have total cholesterol (TC) levels which carry at least a twofold risk of major CHD. Only one third of all the heart attacks occur in the 20% of men with the highest level of TC. The most effective way of reducing morbidity and mortality from CHD would be to move the population

Strategies for Prevention in General Practice.

Population Strategy
- aims to target everybody in the practice

High Risk Strategy
- aims to identify and target only individual patients at high risk

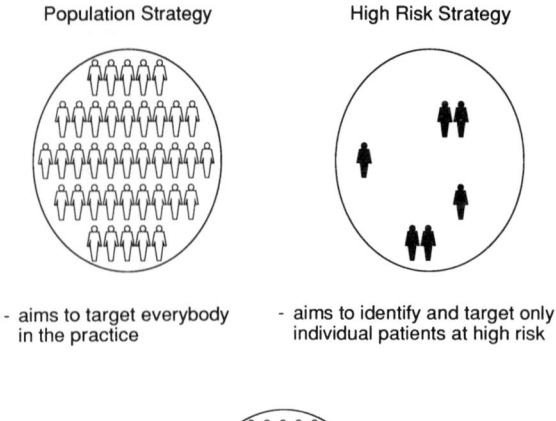

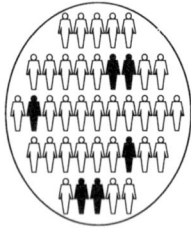

A combination of both strategies is best for a general practice population

Fig. 5.3 Strategies for prevention in general practice.

mean cholesterol level to the left, thus reducing the risk of the majority. In the case of cholesterol this would be mainly by dietary means, i.e. reducing the proportion of calories from saturated fat. This is most likely to be achieved by public health measure, e.g. general health education, food and pricing policy, labelling of foods, etc.

Another example of a population strategy is the reduction of alcohol-related morbidity and mortality. Reducing the number of people drinking at moderate risk levels (14–35 units/week in women and 21–50 units in men) would have a greater effect than identifying and offering treatment to those drinking at harmful levels(>35 units for women >50 units for men).

Whilst public health measures — e.g. dietary recommendations, raising the taxes on cigarettes and alcohol — are the most effective population strategies at a national level, the population strategy has a part to play in prevention at a practice level. For example, it is appropriate to give everybody in a practice dietary advice aimed at reducing serum cholesterol, as it may be safely assumed that everybody has a level which carries some risk of coronary heart disease.

Table 5.1 Advantages and disadvantages of the two prevention strategies

	Population strategy	High-risk strategy
1. Advice tailored to the individual	−	+
2. Subject motivated	−	+
3. Physician motivated	−	+
4. Major benefit to individual	−	+
5. Major benefit to population	+	−
6. Cost-effective use of resources	+	−
7. Benefit – risk ratio	−	+

+ = advantage of one over the other.

The *high-risk* individual approach comes more naturally to the clinician. This approach aims to identify and treat individuals with a high risk of developing a disease (e.g. those with familial hypercholesterolaemia, individuals with high alcohol consumption). In a general practice a combination of these two approaches is desirable, i.e. dietary advice to everybody in the practice with screening and, when indicated, specific treatment (e.g. with lipid lowering drugs) of those at particularly high risk. The population and high-risk approaches to prevention are compared in Table 5.1.

Summary

1. The aims of disease prevention and health promotion are to give 'years to life' and 'life to years'.
2. The key areas for prevention identified in *The Health of the Nation* are coronary heart disease and stroke, cancers, mental illness, HIV/AIDS and sexual health and accidents.
3. The primary health care team has an important role to play in the preventive care of both 'high-risk' individuals and the whole practice population.

Screening

A wide range of screening procedures are carried out in general practice (see box below). The possibility of being able to detect and treat presymptomatic disease and thus prevent or at least reduce its morbidity and mortality has, in the past, generated considerable enthusiasm. The finding of hidden morbidity amongst the people screened at the Peckham pioneer health centre and the description by Last (1963) of the 'iceberg of disease' provided the impetus to an expansion of screening activities.

More recently, as we shall see later in this chapter, the enthusiasm has been tempered by a more critical approach to screening.

What is screening?

Screening is synonymous with secondary prevention and can be defined as the questioning, examination or investigation of an asymptomatic individual to determine the presence or absence of disease.

A screening test is not intended to be diagnostic. It is used to sort out apparently well persons who appear to have the disease which is being screened for, from those who probably do not have the disease.

Screening procedures in general practice

Antenatal screening
- Down's syndrome
- Neural tube defects
- Syphilis
- Rubella

Neonatal
- Phenylketonuria
- Congenital hypothyroidism
- Congenital dislocation of the hip
- Undescended testes
- Heart disease
- Developmental disorders

Childhood
- Immunisation status
- Visual/hearing impairment
- Mental and physical development

Adults
- Risk factors for coronary heart disease and stroke
  — Cigarette smoking
  — Alcohol consumption
  — Blood cholesterol level
  — Blood pressure
  — Weight
- For women
  — Cervical cancer
  — Breast cancer

Old age
- Sight and hearing
- Mobility
- Mental state
- Anaemia
- Blood pressure

Various screening strategies have been described and the terminologies used may lead to confusion. Some commonly used definitions are:

- *Population* or *mass screening* applies to a screening procedure which is offered to a whole population.
- *Multiple* or *multiphasic screening* is when a variety of screening tests are carried out at the same time. This type of screening is often adopted by the private health care organisations offering screening packages.
- *Selective screening* is the offering of a screening procedure to selected groups in a population which are considered to have an increased risk of having the condition, e.g. mammography for women aged over 50 years.
- *Surveillance* is the long-term observation of individuals or population, e.g. developmental screening for preschool children.
- *Case finding* is the screening of patients already in contact with the health services and is the same as opportunistic screening. The contact, but not always the screening activity, is usually patient initiated.

Important characteristics of all types of screening are that the person being screened is asymptomatic for the condition being sought and that the intervention is usually initiated by the doctor. Ideally the person or team responsible for the care of the individual should carry out the screening procedure. Any intervention or treatment which is required is then an integral part of the individual's overall care. Screening carried out by a group or organisation which does not have responsibility of the overall care of the individual is an example of the separation of prevention from care and cure.

Why carry out screening?

The majority of screening procedures carried out in general practice aim to improve the health and life expectancy of the individual patient. The term *prescriptive screening* is often used in this context. Screening may be carried out in the interest of people other than the patient. The best example of this is screening of contacts of a patient found to have tuberculosis. Pre-employment screening and routine examinations for insurance purposes were the earliest examples of screening.

What conditions should be screened for?

The criteria which should be fulfilled before screening for a particular condition is adopted have been defined by Wilson and Jungner (quoted in Holland & Stewart 1990) and are given below.

1. The condition should be an *important health problem*.
2. The *natural history* of the disease should be adequately understood.
3. There should be a *recognisable latent* or *early symptomatic stage*.

4. There should be a *suitable test or examination*, i.e. simple to perform and interpret, acceptable to those taking part, accurate and repeatable, and sensitive and specific.
5. Treatment started at an early stage should be of more benefit than treatment started at a later stage.
6. There should be *accepted treatment* for patients with recognised disease.
7. There should be an agreed policy on who should receive treatment.
8. Diagnosis and treatment should be cost-effective.
9. Case finding should be a continuing process.

These criteria will be discussed in relation to a specific screening procedure later in this chapter. Assessment of the suitability of the screening test (criterion 4.) requires an understanding of test characteristics and will be discussed in the next section.

Screening test characteristics

Ideally a screening test should select only those people who, on further testing, are found to have the disease (i.e. it should have 100% sensitivity). All people without the disease should produce a negative screening test (i.e. the test should be 100% specific). In reality the ideal test does not exist, as we shall see by considering the specificity, sensitivity and predictive power of a screening test in greater detail.

The sensitivity of a screening test (e.g. the cervical smear) is the ability of a test to identify correctly those individuals who have the disease, as determined by a reference test (e.g. cone biopsy). It is a measure of the *true positive rate*. A highly sensitive test will have a *low false negative rate*.

The specificity of a screening test is the ability of the test to identify correctly those who do not have the disease. It is a measure of the *true negative rate*. A highly specific test will have *a low false positive* rate.

The other important characteristics of a test are its positive and negative predictive values.

The *positive predictive value* is the proportion of patients with a positive screening test who actually have the disease.

The *negative predictive value* is the proportion of patients who screen negative who do not have the disease.

The method of calculating the sensitivity, specificity and predictive values of a screening test is shown in Table 5.2.

It is important to understand that the predictive value of a test depends on the *prevalence* of the disease (i.e. the total number of cases in a population) which is being screened for. If a disease is common in the population which is being screened, then the proportion of true positives is greater than when the prevalence is low.

Table 5.2 Calculation of the sensitivity, specificity and predictive values of a screening test

Screening test *Positive*	Reference test *Negative*	*Totals*
Positive a	b	(a+b)
Negative c	d	(c+d)
Totals (a+c)	(b+d)	

False +ves = b
Sensitivity = $\frac{a}{a+c}$
+ve predictive value = $\frac{a}{a+b}$

False −ves = c
Specificity = $\frac{d}{b+d}$
−ve predictive value = $\frac{d}{c+d}$

Critical evaluation of screening procedures

At a time when screening activities are increasing in general practice, it is appropriate to step back and look critically at two of the most common screening procedures carried out in general practice, i.e. cervical screening and general health checks.

Cervical screening Cervical cytology is one of the most common screening procedures carried out in this country, with an increasing number of smears being carried out in general practice. Screening for cervical cancer was introduced in the 1960s before it was properly evaluated. The ideal method of demonstrating the effectiveness of a screening procedure is by carrying out a randomised controlled trial such as the mammography trials carried out in Sweden and the United States. No such trials have been or ever will be carried out for cervical screening.

Evidence has accumulated from other sources that a well-organised screening programme does lead to a reduction in mortality from cervical cancer. The screening programmes in Finland, Iceland and Sweden have covered 80% of women between 25 and 60 years and have achieved reductions in mortality of 50% or more. The situation is different in Denmark and Norway where the screening programmes have reached only 35% and 3% of the target population respectively and there has been a much smaller reduction in mortality — 25% in Denmark and only 2% in Norway. In the United Kingdom the number of smears taken has increased dramatically from 700 000 in 1965 to 4 000 000 in 1985, but this has not been accompanied by a significant decline in mortality. This has been attributed to a poorly organised screening programme with smears being repeated at too frequent intervals in young, low-risk women, inaccurate age-sex registers, failure to reach the women at greatest risk and inadequate follow-up of women with abnormal smears. Another possible reason for the observed failure of mortality from cervical cancer to decline is an increased incidence of carcinoma in situ and invasive carcinoma. There is evidence of an increase in the rate of positive smears taken from women aged 35 and under. Also the number of cases of carcinoma in situ registered in women aged 25–35 increased by 131% between 1973 and 1980. This perhaps reflects the declining use of barrier methods of contraception.

Another way of evaluating a screening programme is to look at the extent to which it satisfies Wilson and Jungner's criteria.

Is cervical cancer an important health problem? This can be assessed by looking at the incidence and mortality of the disease. In 1984 8500 women were found to have carcinoma in situ and 4000 had invasive carcinoma: 1 900 women died from the disease and, of these, 94% were aged over 35. However, it is not a major cause of death in women, accounting for 3% of all female cancer deaths; breast cancer kills ten times more women each year, 20% of all cancer deaths in women.

Is the natural history understood? Cervical cancer is almost certainly caused by the human papilloma virus (HPV), of which there are many types which appear to vary in oncogenic potential. HPV types 16 and 18 have been found to be present in over 80% of invasive squamous carcinomas of the cervix and CIN III intra-epithelial neoplasia in one study; types 6 and 8 were found to be associated with benign warts or mild dysplasia. The natural history of the disease is less well understood. The time taken to progress from CIN I to invasive carcinoma is uncertain because the evidence is difficult to acquire. Many women with invasive carcinoma (66% in one study) have never had a smear and therefore the time taken for progression cannot be determined. Those women who are found to have CIN I and II are usually cured by treatment. It is known that some women who have had repeated smears have shown rapid progression from CIN I to invasive carcinoma.

Is there a recognisable early stage? The answer to this is obviously yes. Cervical intra-epithelial neoplasia and carcinoma in situ can be diagnosed histologically and treated before progression to invasive carcinoma occurs.

Is there a suitable screening test? The taking of a cervical smear is, in principle, easy to perform and interpret. However, there is a significant false negative rate and there are several reasons for this. Studies have shown that general practitioners, gynaecologists and nurses vary in their ability to obtain adequate smears and that cytologist do not always agree on their grading of cell samples. In addition, some women with cervical dysplasia may not produce sufficient abnormal cells to produce a positive smear and in older women the transformation zone moves into the os, which may only be reached by the endo-cervical brush or a spatula with an extended tip.

The sensitivity and specificity of the cervical smear test have been estimated using colposcopy as the reference test. It was concluded that the test has a sensitivity of 80% (i.e. it correctly identifies 80% of those who have the disease and therefore has a *false negative* rate of 20%). The specificity of the test is much higher at 98.5%, i.e. *false positives* rarely occur.

How acceptable is the test? Some women do not attend for cervical screening. This may be for practical reasons, e.g. they do not receive the invitation because it is incorrectly addressed. Others may not attend because they do not accept the need to be tested or may find the test embarrassing. There may be lack of understanding about the test and the disease, e.g. patients may associate the test with promiscuity and decide that they do not need to be tested or they may not realise the need for continued monitoring. Embarrassment at having an internal examination performed may deter some women, particularly if female personnel are not available to perform the test. It has been suggested that if patients' practical, education and emotional needs are met, only about 10% of women will refuse to attend for cervical screening.

DISCUSSION POINT

Screening procedures

Discuss Wilson and Jungner's criteria in relation to another screening procedure commonly carried out in general practice.

General health checks The idea that morbidity and mortality can be reduced by regular screening of individuals for asymptomatic disease and treating the condition detected is an attractive one. The periodic health examination is widely accepted as beneficial in North America and among some social and occupational groups in this country. What is the evidence that such checks are beneficial?

The only large scale trial of multiphasic screening in this country was carried out by the South London Screening Group in the 1970s. 7000 people aged between 40 and 64 were allocated to either the screening group or control group and were then followed for up to eight years. The screening tests included a chest X-ray, blood tests, faecal occult bloods, blood pressure, vision and hearing, and the results were reported to each person's GP. It was found that 50% of the abnormalities were already known to the general practitioner. Follow-up studies showed no difference either in the mortality of the screened and control groups or in indicators of morbidity including consultation and hospital admission rates. A similar study in the USA carried out by the Kaiser Permanente Group produced similar results. Many general practitioners doubt the value of patients having regular health checks and their scepticism is backed up by the results of these trials.

Whilst there is no evidence that multiphasic screening is beneficial, there is evidence that certain screening procedures commonly carried out in general practice do confer benefit. Fowler & Mant (1990) have identified these as screening for smoking habit, alcohol consumption, hypertension, cervical and breast cancer.

Summary

1. A screening test aims to identify a disease or its precursor in an asymptomatic individual. It is not a diagnostic test.

2. Screening programmes should be carefully evaluated before introducing them in practice.

Health education

One of the most important roles of the primary health care team is as educators — providing patients with information and support which enable them to make appropriate choices for healthy living. Other agencies are involved in health education including government, schools, local health promotion units and the media. In general practice health education activities must reinforce the work of these other agencies. The areas in which health education is most likely to be given in general practice are:

- helping patients to avoid disease and to promote their wellbeing, e.g. providing dietary advice, sensible drinking, how to stop smoking
- helping patients to understand the importance of taking up the offer of screening procedures
- helping patients who have established disease to adopt behaviours which reduce disability
- educating patients about the appropriate use of health service resources.

Some theoretical concepts

Rosenstock's Health Belief Model Traditionally the focus of health education has been on providing patients with information, expecting this to increase their knowledge and lead to a change in their beliefs, attitudes and health-related behaviours. However, this sequence is rarely followed and we now realise that helping patients to change involves more than just providing information. Our understanding of how we can help patients to change their behaviour has been helped by the health belief model which was originally formulated in the 1950s by Rosenstock, an American social psychologist. The Rosenstock model describes five factors which help to determine a person's health beliefs. These are:

- The *motivation* of the individual to look after their health
- How they perceive their *vulnerability* to a particular disease
- How they perceive the *seriousness* of the consequences of developing a particular disease or leaving it untreated.
- How they view the physical, psychological and social *cost and benefit* of a particular course of action

- The *cues to action* they receive from either external sources such as newspaper articles or advice from friends or from internal sources such as the development of a symptom.

The model can be summarised as the 3 Ss:

- perceived *S*usceptibility
- perceived *S*eriousness of the disease threat
- viable *S*olutions proposed.

Rosenstock's work helps us not only to develop ways of providing effective health education (as we shall see later in this section) but also to predict compliance behaviour.

Approaches to health education There are three approaches to health education:
- disease-orientated
- risk-factor-orientated
- health-orientated.

In *disease-orientated* health education there is a focus on a particular disease, e.g. cardiovascular disease, and the action is focused on the risk factors, e.g. providing dietary advice. The problem with this approach is that there is an overlap in risk factors for many types of disease (e.g. smoking for coronary heart disease and lung cancer), and the orientation is expert dominated, the expert (the doctor) focusing on an area of her expertise (disease) and imparting information to the patient. The focus is a negative one, emphasising prevention of disease rather than promotion of health.

An alternative approach is to focus attention and action on *risk factors* rather than on the associated disease, e.g. focusing on smoking as a risk factor for carcinoma of the lung and coronary heart disease. This process recognises that single risk factors can be linked to more than one disease and therefore there is less duplication. But the approach is still expert dominated and the emphasis is again on disease prevention rather than health promotion.

The *health-orientated* approach focuses attention and action on behaviour which contributes to positive health and prevents ill-health. For example, it can be pointed out that a healthy diet can be enjoyable, contributing to wellbeing in a positive way rather than just being a way of preventing diseases.

Health education is about helping individuals to adopt behaviours which promote health. We must remember that the decision to change belongs to the patient and that their ability to change depends not only on their motivation and their individual skills, but also on their environment. However well motivated an individual is, it is undoubtedly more difficult to follow a healthy life style if they have an inadequate income, bad housing and work in a dangerous environment. In providing health education we are aiming to help people to take control over decisions that affect their health, not simply providing information and expecting a change in behaviour.

Health education in practice

Health education involves exchanging (not just giving) information. This means that there must be good and effective channels of communication between the patient and the person involved in providing health education. Effective communication — using the skills of active listening, open questioning and picking up verbal and non-verbal cues — is essential. In addition, there is evidence that patients' recall of information given during a consultation is significantly improved if some simple rules are followed. Thus, when providing health education:

- Use short words and short sentences.
- Organise the information into clear categories.
- Give instructions and advice *early* in the interview.
- Stress the *importance* of the advice and the instructions you give.
- *Repeat* the advice during the course of the interview.
- Give *specific* advice.

Besides using good communication skills, it is essential when giving information to ensure that there is an exchange of information and ideas between patient and educator. A *health education interview* can be conveniently divided into four phases:

- *Elicit* the person's health beliefs. Rosenstock's model is helpful in exploring these beliefs.
- *Information phase.* This is a two-way process with the educator seeking information from the patient and at the same time providing information.
- *Negotiating phase.* If the patient decides to make a change then an achievable and realistic target must be discussed, choices offered and action agreed. The desirability for continued support is then discussed.
- *Promoting change.* Ways of promoting change include support from family and friends, ways in which the individual can recognise the achievement by rewarding himself, and perhaps general changes in life style.

Ideally, health education should be part of every consultation but may be limited by the time available. The study of the process and content of consultations of varying length, which was carried out by Morrell et al (1986), found that general practitioners were more likely to give health education advice in the longer (10-minute) than in the shorter (5-minute) consultation. Practice nurses play an important part in providing health education and may be more effective because they may have more time available and the patient may feel more comfortable discussing their life style with the nurse. Training in health education techniques should be provided for staff carrying out this important role.

Studies have shown that reinforcing the verbal advice with appropriate pamphlets helps the patient to retain information and make choices. Health education resources including pamphlets and videos are usually available from local health promotion units.

Summary

1. Health education involves more than giving information: it is helping people to take control over decisions that affect their health.
2. An understanding of a patient's health beliefs and the ability to communicate and negotiate with them are essential skills in health education.

The ethics of prevention and health promotion

In prevention, just as in the treatment of disease, we have a duty to ensure that the benefit of the procedure outweighs any possible harm to the patient, to respect the patient's autonomy and to distribute our resources fairly. It is particularly important to follow these basic ethical principles in preventive activities when it is usually the doctor, rather than the patient, who initiates the activity.

Screening

Whilst screening is beneficial to the individual patient who is found to have a disease, it is important to be aware of the potential harmful effects of screening procedures. False positive results, e.g. the finding of a suspicious lesion on a mammogram which subsequently is shown to be benign, can lead to considerable anxiety for a woman while waiting for diagnostic tests; false negative results may be equally harmful. It has been shown that the 'labelling' of patients with a diagnosis of hypertension which is borderline, has a significant negative effect on their psychological health. During screening programmes patient autonomy should be respected — a particularly difficult and sensitive issue when practices are set screening targets to achieve. Mant & Fowler (1990) suggested that when setting up screening programmes the following points should be considered:

- Inform each patient of the balance of risk and benefit of the screening procedure.
- Ensure that the screening procedure is of high quality and therefore minimise the number of false positive and false negative results.
- Ensure that the intervention offered is effective.
- Routinely audit the completeness of follow-up.

Health education

There is a temptation to consider this as being entirely beneficial and not to look for possible harmful effects. However, health education may also provoke anxiety in patients and some feel that it promotes self-concern which may be damaging. Some of the behaviour which is promoted, e.g. a low-fat diet for patients with raised cholesterol, may itself have harmful effects as some recent studies have hinted. The autonomy of patients must be respected when providing health education — information can be provided and exchanged with the individual patient but the decision whether or not to accept the advice is theirs and theirs alone.

Another concern which has been voiced about health promotion activities in primary care is the effect on the doctor/patient relationship. For example, failing to recognise the patient's right to refuse to have a cervical smear may result in excessive pressure being placed on the woman and may deter her from consulting in the future. The use of resources should also be considered — for example, holding health promotion clinics may reduce the time available for other activities, which may be considered to be more important in the practice.

DISCUSSION POINTS

Health education

A case history for discussion:

Mrs A smokes 20 cigarettes a day and presents *to you with* an upper respiratory tract infection. She is separated from her husband and copes alone with three small children. 'Smoking is my only pleasure', she says. Discuss the issues involved in advising Mrs A about her smoking habits.

You decide to set up a well person clinic in your practice. Discuss the ways by which you would ensure that the benefit to patients is maximised and the harm minimised.

DISEASE PREVENTION AND HEALTH PROMOTION IN PRACTICE

In the first part of this chapter we have looked at some of the theoretical concepts which are important in our understanding of how we can help in preventing disease and promoting the health of our patients. In the remainder of this chapter we shall look at the ways in which the theories can be put into practice by considering some of the preventive activities carried out in general practice.

Why is general practice considered to be the ideal setting for preventing disease and promoting health? The reasons can be grouped under three headings.

1. *Patient contact*
   - The majority of patients (95%) visit their general practitioner at least once every 3 years and 70% consult at least once a year.
   - The continuing contact with patients is important so that health education messages can be reinforced and uptake of screening procedures monitored.
   - The fact that whole families are usually registered with a practice can be very useful in discussing prevention issues.
2. *The doctor/patient relationship.* The continuing, potentially life-long relationship and the trust which patients place in their doctors is important. Patients expect doctors to be interested in their life style and to give appropriate advice.
3. *The practice team.* Prevention is a team effort because of the different skills required. Practice nurses are becoming increasingly involved in disease prevention/health promotion, and staff with other skills, e.g. counsellors, are becoming members of the primary health care team.

Practice organisation

An efficient records system and motivated trained staff are essential for an effective programme of prevention/health promotion in a practice.

Records

An accurate age/sex register is vital and this must be kept up-to-date. With increasing computerisation in practices it has become easier to ensure accuracy. When FHSAs produce age/sex registers, these need to be checked against practice records.

The format of patients' records is also important. Information about life style habits and uptake of screening procedures needs to be up-to-date and readily accessible when the patient consults. This is most easily done when records are computerised and the computer can be used to produce a surgery list with prompts about preventive activities which need to be carried out, e.g. Mrs Smith; Cx smear. Prevention cards have been designed on which relevant up-to-date information can be recorded and kept in a prominent position in a patient's notes (Fig. 5.4) (Grundy & Dwyer 1989). These have been shown to improve recording of risk factors and screening procedures. In some practices family prevention cards have been used and have been found to be useful in deprived populations (Marsh & Channing 1988).

PREVENTIVE CARE CARD

Surname	Forenames		D.o.B.
NHS Number	Blood Group	Height	Male / Female
Allergies/Risk Factors			

IMMUNISATIONS: Enter date and batch number in each box

	1st	2nd	3rd	Pre-School	15+
Pertussis					
Diphtheria					
Tetanus					
Polio					
Measles		Heaf Test	Date Result	BCG	
Rubella		Adult Tetanus			
Mumps					

Additional Immunisations: Enter date, vaccine (or test) and batch number in each box

PREVENTION

B.P.	Date Result					
	Date Result					
SMOKING	Date Result					
ALCOHOL	Date Result					
CERVICAL SMEAR	Date Result					
	Date Result					
RUBELLA STATUS	Date Result					
URINALYSIS	Date Result					
WEIGHT	Date Result					
	Date Result					

Additional Information

	Date Result					
	Date Result					
	Date Result					
	Date Result					

Fig. 5.4 The front and back of a preventive care card. (Published by courtesy of the Joint Working Party of the Tamar Faculty of the RCGP and the Devon and Cornwall LMC.)

Recording sheets for use with patients with specific chronic disorders — e.g. asthma, diabetes and hypertension — have been developed and their use is increasing with the advent of disease monitoring clinics. Patient-held cards may be used in shared care schemes between practices and local hospitals. They provide easily accessible information and reinforce the involvement of patients in their own care.

Practice staff

'Think prevention' is a good motto for all practice staff. The practice nurse is a key figure in preventive activities but should be adequately trained. Many training courses are now available particularly in the management of chronic conditions, e.g. asthma and diabetes. Prevention should be a team effort and it is not appropriate to expect a practice nurse to write a clinic protocol and conduct a clinic by herself. The practice manager, receptionist and practice secretary are increasingly involved with preventive activities particularly since the advent of health promotion clinics. Once again motivation and training are essential.

Facilitators

Facilitators assist practices in the setting up of preventive activities and in the training of practice staff. The first ones were appointed in the Oxford region where a controlled trial showed that practices with a facilitator improved their recording over a 2-year-period of patients' blood pressure from 35% to 59%, smoking habits from 11% to 49% and weight from 12% to 45% (Fullard et al 1987).

Attached staff

Midwives play a major role in practice antenatal clinics, and health visitors act in the preventive care of children and, in some areas, the elderly. The role of district nurses in prevention is less obvious, but in their care of the chronic sick they are exercising a preventive role.

Promoting health in childhood

The opportunities for preventing ill-health and promoting good health in childhood are great and are increasingly being given to the primary health care team. Immunisation, child health surveillance and health education for parents and children are three important areas of anticipatory care. Health in childhood is shaped by influences acting before birth and this underlines the importance of preconception counselling and good antenatal care. Socioeconomic factors are also important: these were discussed earlier in the chapter.

Child health surveillance

General practitioners have become increasingly involved in child health surveillance in recent years, and this is recognised in the statement of fees and allowances, with an allocation of £10 per annum for each child under the age of 5 years on the GP's list. The recommended preschool developmental surveillance programme (Hall 1991) starts with the 6-week neonatal check and ends with the preschool examination when the child is aged 4½ years. General practitioners and health visitors carry out this screening programme.

The aims of a child health surveillance programme have been stated by Bain (1990) to be:

1. to confirm normality and offer guidance on child growth and development
2. to identify variations and deviations from normal development
3. to identify and follow up children with potentially handicapping conditions
4. to provide opportunities for parents to discuss their children's development and health needs.

A child health surveillance programme should not be limited to screening for abnormalities but must include health education as an important part of the programme.

Health education topics for discussion with parents
• Nutrition
• Immunisation uptake
• Accident prevention
• Recognition and management of illness
• Management of behavioural problems
• Hazards of passive smoking

Developing and sustaining the current routine surveillance programme has considerable resource implications for both general practice and the community child health service, to which children who screen positive are referred.

Organisation of CHS in the practice Child health surveillance in general practice is usually carried out in clinics but may be done opportunistically, particularly in deprived areas. The essential features of a successful CHS programme are:

1. An agreed *practice policy* for CHS, see box below.
2. An accurate *age/sex register*.
3. *Facilities and equipment*, i.e. a separate room, toys and books, etc., to make a friendly atmosphere.
4. *Motivated trained staff*. Good teamwork, particularly with midwives and health visitors, is essential, General practitioners must provide evidence of their competence to carry out CHS before admission to the approved list held by FHSAs entitling them to payment. The criteria for admission to the list vary between FHSAs. Evidence of proficiency in CHS is now required before admission to the MRCGP examination which entitles the holder to enter the CHS list. Attendance at refresher courses is required by most FHSAs.
5. *An organised records system*. Data for each child are now held on a centralised computer system within each district (The child health computing system). There is a move to 'parent-held' child health records which have been shown to be acceptable to health visitors, doctors and parents and which reinforce the parents' role in promoting their children's health.

Practice policy for child surveillance

1. A shared team commitment to the surveillance of children.
2. A clearly defined surveillance programme with agreed allocation of responsibilities within the team.
3. An up-to-date record of all children under 5 years in the practice.
4. Surveillance clinics kept separate from the routine care of sick children (to avoid confusion for parents about the role and function of child health surveillance clinics).
5. Continuous monitoring of performance.
6. Regular contact between doctors, health visitors, and other practice staff involved in organising preschool examinations.

(After Bain 1990)

Evaluation of child health surveillance This is difficult. Some critics of the programme have questioned its cost-effectiveness, pointing out that many of the procedures are of unproven value and that parents are best placed to identify and report possible abnormalities or problems which require further assessment. An additional difficulty is that there are no fixed points in a child's development which offer clear-cut distinctions between normality and abnormality, e.g. most late developers in walking turn out to be normal. Monitoring of CHS has been carried out in Northumberland using available data sets and the following outcome measures (Colver 1990):

1. Proportion of eligible children immunised and screened

2. Age at diagnosis and treatment of congenital deafness, cerebral palsy and special educational needs.

> **DISCUSSION POINT**
>
> **Child health surveillance**
>
> — How would you evaluate the CHS programme in a practice?

Immunisation

Immunisation is the best example of primary prevention carried out in general practice. For the majority of vaccines it is of proven cost-effectiveness. Immunisation programmes lead to a fall in the number of notified cases of a disease, the number of deaths and, particularly in the case of rubella, long-term sequelae. This relationship is shown for whooping cough in Figure 5.5. Other diseases, e.g. measles, have followed a similar pattern after the introduction of the vaccine. The graph for whooping cough shows an increase in the number of cases in the late 1970s and reflects the fall in immunisation uptake to 31% in 1978, due largely to parental anxiety about the safety of the vaccine. The subsequent public education campaign was successful and uptake has more than doubled since 1978, reaching 75% in England and Wales in 1988/9.

The World Health Organization set out its aims to eliminate measles, polio, diphtheria, tetanus in the newborn and congenital rubella by the year 2000, and these aims were adopted by the Department of Health. A target

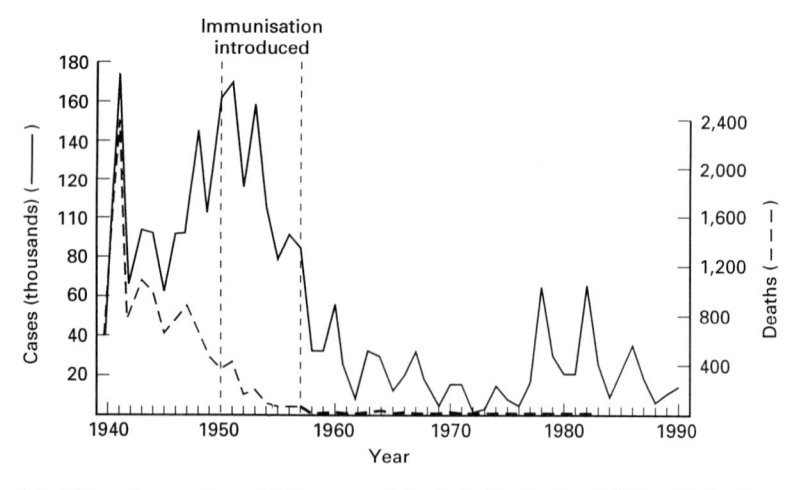

Fig. 5.5 Whooping cough: notified cases and deaths in England and Wales, 1940–90. Source: OPCS. (Published by courtesy of the Royal College of Physicians of London 1991.)

of 90% immunisation uptake rates was set for each of these diseases in children under 2 years and the target was to achieve this uptake by 1990. Although it is recognised that total eradication of these diseases may not be possible, reaching 90% uptake rates should be achievable and an upward trend in uptake has been recorded in Britain.

The link between remuneration and target levels achieved in general practice, which was introduced in the 1990 Contract, and the revision of the immunisation policy (have contributed to the rise in uptake. The immunisation) of babies at an earlier age — at two, three and four months — is not only effective but enables the programme to be linked more closely with the timing of child health surveillance. The introduction of the measles, mumps, rubella (MMR) vaccine has significantly improved the level of protection against measles and rubella, for which individual vaccines were previously available. The congenital rubella syndrome (CRS) is one of a few congenital problems that is, in principle, totally preventable. Immunisation of girls aged 10–13 was introduced in the early 1970s, as was immunisation of all non-pregnant women of child-bearing age who were not immune. However, cases of CRS still occur and it is hoped that the syndrome will be totally eliminated in future years because of the MMR vaccine.

The role of the primary health care team in maximising immunisation uptake rates is vital. Good organisation within the practice, an efficient record system and the involvement and education of parents are particularly important. Six factors which are important in achieving maximum uptake are shown below.

Key features of successful immunisation programme
1. An organised, computerised call and recall system.
2. A motivated primary health care team.
3. A strategy for reaching socially deprived and highly mobile groups.
4. Education of parents and professionals about the benefits of immunisation.
5. Good liaison between district health authorities, practice staff and parents.
6. Regular audit with feedback to practices.

Summary

1. Health promotion in childhood involves:
    - Immunisation
    - Child health surveillance
    - Health education.
2. Parents must be involved and their concerns must be heard and taken seriously.

Promoting a healthy life style

The link between life style, disease and premature death is well established. One of the most important roles of the GP and other members of the primary health care team is to help patients to adopt a healthy life style.

Smoking

One hundred thousand people die each year in Britain from smoking-related diseases. The majority die from lung cancer, chronic obstructive airways disease and coronary heart disease. Smoking is related to a number of other diseases and, in pregnant women, it is a serious hazard to the baby. It is the single most preventable cause of death. The cost of smoking is outlined below.

The cost of smoking

- In Britain smoking accounts for 100 000 deaths/year:
  - 90% of the 40 000 lung cancer deaths
  - 75% of the 20 000 deaths from chronic obstructive lung disease
  - 25% of the 180 000 deaths from coronary artery disease.
- Passive smoking causes 1000 deaths/year.
- NHS services for patients with smoking-related diseases cost £500 million each year.

(Royal College of Physicians of London 1991)

A study of smoking trends shows that smoking has declined since the 1950s, particularly amongst the professional classes. However, figures from the 1988 General Household Survey showed that 33% of men and 30% of women were cigarette smokers. Decline in smoking has been less steep amongst women and there has been a slight increase in the number of young women smoking. Amongst children and adolescents, 28% have tried a cigarette before the age of 10, and 7% of boys and 9% of girls in the age range 11–15 are regular smokers. Smoking is most prevalent in the lower socioeconomic classes.

Smoking is one of the top priorities of the Government's white paper *Health of the Nation:* the target is to reduce the proportion of men smoking cigarettes to 22% and of women to 21% by the year 2000. How is this going to be achieved? The *Health of the Nation* document emphasises the role of the primary health care team. However, government itself must play a major role in helping us to achieve the target set. An increase in tax on tobacco would have a major impact together with controls on promotion in the media and control of smoking in public places. These are prevention strategies working at the *population* level. Other population strategies include prominent health warnings on cigarette packets, banning the sale of cigarettes to children and greater emphasis on health education both in schools and in the community.

The role of the primary health care team At least a quarter of a million smokers consult their general practitioner each day and studies have shown that the majority expect the doctor to enquire about their life style and to give appropriate advice. Several studies have shown that with minimal intervention (advice and a leaflet) general practitioners can help about 5% of their smokers to stop smoking. This figure rises when more effective methods including use of Nicorette and the setting up of special clinics are used. It has been calculated that general practitioners in this country could help 500 000 smokers a year to stop smoking.

What strategies can we use to reduce smoking in our practice population? They include:

1. Health education for children and adolescents about the hazards of smoking
2. Recording of the smoking habits of all patients in their medical records
3. Helping established smokers to stop by means of opportunistic health education, health education given as part of general health checks and the setting up of Stop Smoking clinics.

In addition, all practices should consider establishing a 'No Smoking' policy in the practice and the use of posters and literature, particularly to coincide with media campaigns such as the 'No Smoking Day'.

How to help someone stop smoking We are in an excellent position to help our patients stop smoking because the help which we give can be highly personalised to the individual. However, stopping smoking is not a sudden single event. It usually involves four stages.

1. The person thinks about stopping — this may be influenced by advertising or increase in cigarette prices, etc.

2. They decide and prepare to stop. A person may stop smoking suddenly because of a smoking-related illness or they may need to develop a strategy or plan, often with the help of a health care professional or self-help literature.

3. They actually stop smoking — support either by friends or a group is important at this stage.

4. Permanently stopping — again support and encouragement are often necessary at this stage to prevent relapse.

Within a consultation (i.e. stage 2) a possible sequence of events is shown below:

- Raise the issue.
- Record smoking habits in medical records.
- Inquire about interest in giving up.

- Give information and advice about stopping.
- Help the person to plan a strategy for stopping.
- Offer written advice, follow-up and support.

Summary

1. Smoking is the single most important cause of death in the western world — and the most preventable.

2. The primary health care team can play a major role in advising about the hazards of smoking and helping people to stop.

Alcohol

Excessive alcohol consumption probably causes, or directly contributes to, at least 40 000 deaths per year in England and Wales. Like smoking, the burden in terms of lives lost, lives impaired and the use of NHS and social services resources is considerable. The financial cost in England and Wales in 1983 has been estimated at £1614.5 million. The importance of government action (in terms of pricing of alcohol, etc.) in reducing this burden is obvious, but action has not been forthcoming. This issue is complex as the country gains £6000 million each year from duty and exports and the alcohol industry employs 250 000 people.

DISCUSSION POINT

Promoting a healthy life style

— What role should doctors play in influencing the tobacco and alcohol policies of government?

The role of the primary health care team Unlike smoking, moderate alcohol consumption is pleasurable and socially acceptable. There is evidence that drinking at a 'safe' level does no harm and some say that it confers benefit, although this is controversial. The task in the practice is therefore to promote *sensible* drinking by:

- Giving appropriate *health education,* including the use of posters and pamphlets, to everybody in the practice
- *Recording drinking habits* (in terms of units/week) of patients in their notes
- *Identifying* those who are drinking at levels which may damage them physically, psychologically and/or socially.

The physical, psychological and social effects of excessive alcohol consumption are well known. The individual patient who is alcohol dependent with cirrhosis, a broken marriage and no job is not difficult to recognise, but usually very difficult to help. The middle-aged businessman or the elderly widow drinking above the safe level in the hazardous range may be difficult to identify but amenable to help. Identification involves a high level of awareness. The simplest and most direct method is to take a person's drinking history as routinely as taking their smoking history. Taking a drinking history involves going over the amount of alcohol consumed during the previous 7 days, day by day. The amount should then be converted to units of alcohol and related to the recommended 'safe' levels of 21 units/week for men and 14 units/week for women.

Converting amounts of alcohol to units

- 1 unit = 8 g of alcohol, contained in:
  — 1 glass of wine
  — ½ pint of beer
  — 1 *pub* measure of spirits

  (N.B. 'Home' measures may contain 3–4 units)

- A guide for LOW-RISK DRINKING is up to:
  — 21 units a week for men
  — 14 units a week for women
  with preferably some drink-free days.

- It is DANGEROUS to drink persistently more than:
  — 50 units a week for men
  — 35 units a week for women

A drinking history can be backed up by asking the patient to complete a screening questionnaire such as the CAGE questionnaire (see below). Blood tests (Gamma GT & MCV) have been used to identify 'problem' drinkers but are less accurate than taking a drinking history or using a questionnaire.

CAGE Questionnaire

1. Have you ever felt you should *cut* down on your drinking?
2. Have people *annoyed* you by criticising your drinking?
3. Have you ever felt bad or *guilty* about your drinking?
4. Have you ever had a drink first thing in the morning (*eye-opener*) to steady your nerves or to get rid of a hangover?
   - A positive response to 3 or 4 items — almost definitely has a serious alcohol problem.
   - 2 items — probably has a serious alcohol problem.
   - 0–1 items — probably does not have an alcohol problem.

Helping a person to change their drinking habits Patients who are alcohol dependent or who are drinking at harmful levels are likely to benefit from referral for specialist help (either within the NHS or to a voluntary agency). Those drinking above the 'safe' level in the 'harmful' range need advice and counselling which should include the following phases:

- *Elicit information* about the person's drinking behaviour and their beliefs and attitudes about alcohol.
- *Give information* about the harmful effects of alcohol and recommended levels of consumption.
- *Negotiate*; having had time to reflect on the information given, the person should be encouraged to make a *choice* about altering his drinking behaviour. This choice must be respected.
- *Goal setting* and *ongoing support* for those who decide to change their drinking behaviour.

Prevention of coronary heart disease

This deserves special attention because coronary heart disease is a major cause of mortality, it is potentially preventable and the primary health care team can play a key role in its prevention (Hart 1990). It provides a model for disease prevention and health promotion in general practice. The concept of risk is central to this discussion and the relevant definitions of risk are given below.

What is risk?

- ABSOLUTE RISK is the chance of something happening, e.g. the risk of dying from a myocardial infarction during the next 5 years for a man aged 52 years.
- RELATIVE RISK compares the risk of an individual or group exposed to a particular risk factor compared with an individual or group not exposed, e.g. the risk of a smoker having a myocardial infarct compared with a non-smoker.
- ATTRIBUTABLE RISK is the amount of disease (e.g. coronary heart disease) which can be attributed to a risk factor (e.g. raised blood cholesterol).

Risk factors for coronary heart disease

These can be classified on the basis of whether or not they can be modified.
— *Unmodifiable risk factors:*
- age
- sex
- family history
- race
- previous history of ischaemic heart disease.

— *Modifiable risk factors:*
- smoking
- raised serum cholesterol
- hypertension
- diabetes
- exercise
- obesity.

These factors have been identified and their relative importance determined in epidemiological studies. An international study (the Seven Countries Study) showed that the most important factor in determining population risk for CHD was the mean serum total cholesterol (TC). If this is low, as it is in Japan, then the prevalence of CHD is low in spite of the fact that the Japanese have high prevalences of smoking and hypertension. Communities with average levels of serum cholesterol in middle-aged men below 5 mmol/1 have a low susceptibility to CHD. In Great Britain, where the mean TC level is 6.3 mmol/1, the level of susceptibility is high. The mean TC level is determined to a large extent by dietary factors, i.e. the ratio of polyunsaturated to saturated fats (p/s ratio) in the usual adult diet. In Japan, where there is low saturated fat intake, the p/s ratio is 1.0 compared with 0.2 in Great Britain.

These studies have also identified factors which *protect* against CHD.

Protective factors for CHD:
1. *Sex.* Young women (35–44 years) are 5–6 times *less* likely to die from CHD than men of the same age. This difference begins to disappear at the time of the menopause.
2. *Physical exercise.* Evidence suggests that regular *moderate* exercise is protective.
3. *High density lipoprotein (HDL) cholesterol level.* High levels appear to confer benefit. It accounts for only one sixth of the TC level and therefore is not a powerful indicator of risk.

Further information on the relationship between the risk factors and the probability of developing CHD has come from two large prospective studies: the Framingham Heart Study in the USA and the British Regional Heart Study. Both studies identified a group of middle-aged people, measured their risk factors and then followed them up over a number of years, recording the recurrence of fatal and non-fatal CHD events. These studies have been able to determine the relative importance of each of the risk factors and the ways in which they interact.

Relative importance of modifiable risk factors Evidence about the relative importance of CHD risk factors and their interaction has come from the British Regional Heart Study (BRHS). This was set up in 1978 and recruited 7735 men aged between 40 and 59 years from general practices in 24 towns in the British Isles. The cardiovascular risk factors of these men were assessed at the start of the study. They have been followed up and the occurrence of fatal and non-fatal heart attacks and strokes has been recorded and linked with the men's risk factors and, in particular, whether they were in the lowest, intermediate or highest part of the distribution, e.g. non-smokers, smoking <20 per day, smoking more than 40 per day.

The findings can be summarized as follows. Each independent risk factor will contribute a 2–3-fold risk gradient across its range of levels.

Where average levels of a risk pertain, such as being an ex-smoker with a TC of 6.0 mmol/l and a systolic blood pressure of 150, the risk conferred is already 10 times greater than a never-smoker with a TC of less than 5.5 mmol/l and a systolic blood pressure of less than 130. The only way to assess multiplicative risk is to use a scientifically based scoring system which provides the best predictive model. One example of a scoring system is the BRHS GP score, which will be discussed later in this chapter.

Effect of risk-factor modification Two types of study have looked at the effect of modifying risk factors in CHD prevalence. One approach has been to focus on whole communities and the other to identify and intervene with high-risk individuals.

Community based programmes Finland has a high mortality rate from cardiovascular disease (CHD, stroke and hypertension), and the North Karalia Project was set up in 1972 in response to this. The community based programme addressed several risk factors and involved both primary and secondary prevention. The incidence of cardiovascular events was compared over a number of years with that in a neighbouring control county where there was no community programme. Follow-up surveys in 1977 and 1982 found that there was a greater reduction in risk factors in North Karalia than in the control county, particularly in cigarette smoking. Between 1974 and 1979 there was a 22% reduction in age-standardised CHD mortality in men in North Karalia compared with 12% in the control county and 11% in the rest of Finland. This, and another community-based study (the WHO European Collaborative Trial), suggests that intervention at a community level can be effective in reducing risk factors and CHD mortality but this is achieved at considerable cost to society.

High-risk programmes The Multiple Risk Factor Intervention Trial (MRFIT), which began in the USA in 1982, is the best known of these studies. Starting with 361 662 men aged between 35 and 57 years, 12 866 were identified who were in the upper range of a risk-score distribution (based on smoking, blood pressure and serum cholesterol level) and who showed no evidence of ischaemic heart disease. Half of this group was allocated to an intervention programme which involved health education and monitoring at 4-monthly intervals. The other half acted as a control group and were seen for an annual medical examination but were not given any advice by the research team. Both the control and intervention groups and their own doctors were given information about their risk-factor status. Over the 7-year follow-up period, smoking, blood pressure and serum TC were decreased in both groups but more so in the intervention group. CHD mortality was reduced by 22% in the intervention group but this was not statistically significant. One reason for this was that the control group had modified their life-style risk factors, probably in response to the information about their individual risk status.

What can be learnt from these and other similar studies?

1. Attempting to change the life style of a community (in terms of reducing CHD risk factors) can lead to a reduction in CHD mortality. However, this involves considerable effort and resources and probably requires a highly motivated community to be successful (as in Finland where CHD mortality is high).

2. Identification of high-risk individuals and the use of intervention programmes to modify their risk factors can lead to a reduction in the CHD mortality.

3. Knowledge of their risk status can motivate some individuals to change their life style.

A strategy for CHD prevention in general practice

The strategy should combine primary, secondary and tertiary prevention. It should adopt both population and high-risk approaches, should involve the whole of the primary health care team and should link with the activities of other health care workers. The health promotion activities which a strategy should encompass are listed below.

Targeting resources A recent study found that three-quarters of patients aged 35–64 need advice or treatment for one or more risk factors and one-third need attention for two or more risk factors. For the average practice this is likely to be a daunting workload. For practices with a high proportion of patients from the lower socioeconomic groups and/or ethnic

---

Strategy for CHD prevention

PRIMARY PREVENTION

- Health education for all
    — Healthy eating
    — Regular exercise
    — No-smoking advice
    — Sensible drinking

SECONDARY PREVENTION

- Screening for individuals at high risk
    — Life-style risk factors
    — Blood pressure
    — Serum cholesterol (when appropriate)

TERTIARY PREVENTION

- Advice to those who have ischaemic heart disease
    — Health education concerning life style

- Medication
    — Aspirin or beta blockers for patients who have had a myocardial infarct (Sometimes called secondary prevention.)

- Rehabilitation
    — Post myocardial infarction

minorities the workload will be even greater. How can we decide where to start and how to target the available resources of the practice?

A working group set up by the Coronary Prevention Group and the British Heart Foundation have made recommendations and developed an action plan for use in general practice (Fig. 5.6). Patients are allocated, on the basis of their medical and family histories, to a *special care group* or a *general advice group*. The latter should receive regular health education and monitoring of any risk factors they have, e.g. borderline hypertension and obesity. This can be done opportunistically or by infrequent recall. The special care group includes those at clinical risk with multiple risk factors and will require extra effort in terms of health education, investigations and

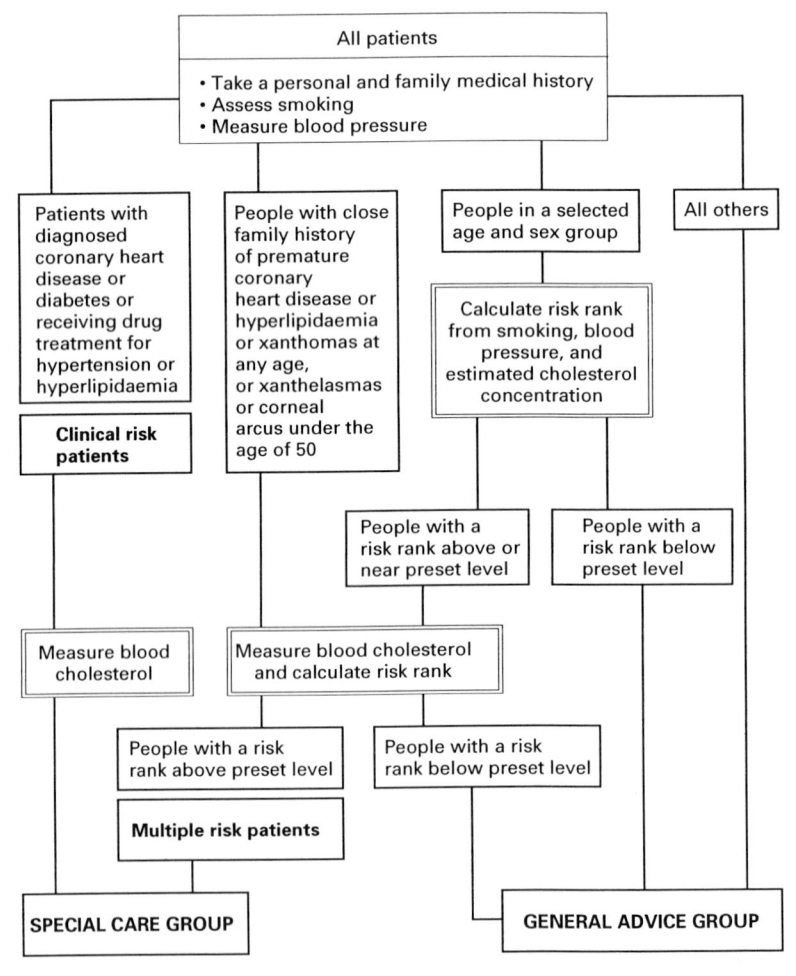

Fig. 5.6 Preventing coronary heart disease in primary care: action plan. (Published by courtesy of the Working Group of the Coronary Prevention Group and the British Heart Foundation 1991.)

monitoring; this may be carried out more effectively in a clinic setting. An important point to note about the plan is that it involves measuring the blood cholesterol of *selected* patients, not of the whole population.

The Coronary Prevention Action plan enables a practice to target its available resources on the group of patients who are likely to benefit most from screening and intervention. How can these patients be identified? At least two methods of scoring an individual's risk have been developed:

1. *The Dundee Risk Score.* The Coronary Prevention Action Plan is based on the Dundee Risk Score which uses three modifiable risk factors, i.e. smoking, blood pressure and blood cholesterol concentration (although for apparently low-risk patients this can be entered initially as an estimated value). An individual's score is calculated using the Dundee coronary risk disc. This expresses the person's risk of having a heart attack over the next five years relative to his or her sex and age group — i.e. it is a measure of *relative* risk. The disc also produces a person's risk rank, i.e. his or her position in a queue of 100 people of the same age and sex. As it is based on modifiable risk factors, a person's rank or position in the queue will change if, for example, they are able to stop smoking. However, it must be stressed that risk will not change immediately as it will take several years for an ex-smoker to return to the risk of a non-smoker.

2. *The British Regional Heart Study (BRHS) GP score.* This is a simple calculation which can be carried out 'by hand' during the consultation. It calculates a patient's *absolute* risk of having a heart attack within the following five years. It is designed for use in general practice as a first-line screening tool. A score of 1000 places a person in the top 20% of the distribution of scores. It is based on smoking history, blood pressure, a personal history of ischaemic heart disease and/or diabetes, chest pain on exertion and a parental death from heart disease. Serum cholesterol is not included as it was found not to significantly increase the predictive value of the score. However, measurement of serum cholesterol should be considered for those identified as high-risk individuals. The method of calculating the score is shown in Table 5.3. Plastic discs to aid the calculation of the score have been developed and it is now part of some software packages.

The BRHS score (also known as the Shaper score) aims to *identify rather than monitor* those individuals at high risk of developing a heart attack who need appropriate health advice, investigation, perhaps medication and certainly follow-up. As the score is predictive it includes several non-modifiable risk factors; it is not used for monitoring change in the person's level of risk. Those factors selected for modification will themselves be the best indicators of change, e.g. smoking, weight, blood pressure.

Use of a risk score Risk assessment enables a practice to identify individuals who require special advice and attention. It is essential that the evaluation and management of risk is negotiated with the individual and takes into account his/her health beliefs and values (remember Rosenstock's Health Belief Model, p. 154). The advice given must be tailored not only to his

Table 5.3 Calculation of British Regional Heart Study GP score

Questions asked in assessment of score

1. How many years have you smoked at least one cigarette daily? _____ x 7.5 =
2. Has a doctor ever told you that you have had angina or heart attack? if YES + 265 =
3. Has a doctor ever told you that you have diabetes? if YES + 150 =
4. Do you ever have any chest pain when walking uphill or hurrying? if YES + 150 =
5. Has either of your parents died of heart trouble? if YES + 80 =
6. Take two blood pressure readings and use average systolic pressure. _____mmHg x 4.5 =

Total =

INTERPRETATION OF SCORE

Risk of having heart attack in five years

For men aged 40–59:

	Score	Risk
High risk	> 1000	1 in 10
	900–999	1 in 25
Average risk	800–899	1 in 30
	700–799	1 in 100
Low risk	< 700	1 in 250
For men aged over 60 Postmenopausal women	A score of 1200 places them in the top 20% high-risk category	

beliefs and attitudes but also to his particular circumstances. The extent to which a person modifies his risk will depend on how he perceives his level of risk, how much he values the outcome and how he perceives the cost-benefits, e.g. of stopping smoking. The use of a risk score can be a motivating force to behavioural change but it can also engender anxiety and negative attitudes to adopting a healthy life style. It can also falsely reassure. Therefore, risk assessment with feedback to the patient, should be carried out with care.

Summary

The prevention of coronary heart disease provides a model for disease prevention and health promotion in general practice.

1. The approach to coronary heart disease prevention must involve primary, secondary and tertiary strategies.
2. The majority of patients in a practice will have one or more risk factors for CHD.

> **DISCUSSION POINTS**
>
> **Prevention of coronary heart disease**
>
> 1. Mr F is a 52-year-old company executive who attends a well person clinic run by your practice nurse. He has smoked 20/day for the past 30 years, is overweight and drinks 40 units of alcohol per week. His blood pressure is 160/100 (mean of 3 readings). His BRHS GP score is 1175. The practice nurse refers him to you for future management as he falls into the highest risk category. Outline what your management might be.
> 2. If Mr F were an unemployed manual worker, would this influence your management plan? If so, how?

3. A practice strategy must combine the population approach (health education for all) with the high risk approach — identifying, intervening and monitoring patients at high risk of CHD.

4. Practice resources are always limited and must be used in the most effective way. This involves setting priorities, e.g. identifying and advising patients at highest risk of developing CHD.

5. Preventive care should be well organised and structured, e.g. practice protocols, methods of recording, recall systems, etc. This applies to whether it is carried out in clinics or within the consultation. Practice staff should be appropriately trained.

6. Special strategies and extra effort may be needed to identify and help those at risk in the lower socioeconomic groups and members of ethnic minorities.

Screening in general practice

In this section we shall look at the prevention of breast cancer and hypertension, with particular emphasis on the role and organisation of screening programmes. These two examples have been chosen to illustrate the part which a general practitioner and team play in a screening programme which takes place outside the practice (breast cancer), and in one which should be practice-based (hypertension). Screening of the elderly is discussed in Chapter 6 (p. 224).

Breast cancer

Breast cancer is the commonest malignancy among women in the UK. One woman in 12 can expect to develop the disease during her lifetime. Each year there are approximately 24 000 new cases and 15 000 women die from the disease. The 5-year survival rate is currently 62%.

The cause of breast cancer is unknown but epidemiological studies have identified a number of risk factors which must be taken into account when planning a prevention strategy.

Risk factors for breast cancer

1. Reproductive factors
   • Nulliparity
   • Age at first pregnancy >35 years
2. Hormonal factors
   • Early menarche
   • Late menopause
3. Social class
   • Women in social class I have twice the risk of those in social class V.
4. Family history
   • Ist degree relative with breast cancer increases risk 2–3 fold.
5. Benign breast disease
   • Women with fibrocystic disease have 2–4 times the risk of developing breast cancer.

Whilst endogenous oestrogens are important in the development of breast cancer, the role of exogenous oestrogens is less certain. As yet there is no conclusive evidence that oral contraceptives or hormone replacement therapy are associated with increased risk, and the results of current trials are awaited. The role of diet is also unclear; there is some evidence that women who have a high-fat, high-calorie, low-fibre diet have an increased risk of developing breast cancer. The association with social class is probably due to the protective effect of the earlier age of first pregnancy of working-class women.

As with most cancers, the incidence rises with age from 19.6/100 000 for women between 30 and 35 years to 145.9/100 000 for women between 50 and 54 years. Thereafter the rate continues to rise with age.

Prevention of breast cancer A review of the risk factors indicates that primary prevention is unlikely to make a significant impact on breast cancer incidence and mortality. There is evidence from clinical trials that prognosis is improved by early diagnosis; this has focused attention and resources on secondary prevention, i.e. methods of screening for breast cancer. Possible screening methods are clinical examination, breast self-examination and mammography. To be effective in reducing breast cancer mortality, screening methods must be able to diagnose tumours before they have spread. In the case of breast cancer there is evidence that these are small tumours of less than 1 cm in diameter. Only mammography has been evaluated in randomised controlled trials, although clinical and self-examination were included in some of these trials. Breast self-examination has been advocated as a screening method. Whilst there is no conclusive evidence that it affects mortality, women should continue to be taught and encouraged to examine their breasts regularly — 90% of *clinically detectable* tumours are identified by the woman herself.

The National Health Service Breast Screening Programme Breast screening by mammography, unlike cervical screening, was introduced only after the results of randomised controlled trials had been evaluated. The two main studies were the New York Health Insurance Plan study in the 1960s and the Swedish two county study in the 1970s. Both studies found a 30% reduction in mortality in the screened population and this was corroborated by case-control studies carried out in Italy and the Netherlands. Based on these findings, the Forrest report, published in 1986, recommended the setting up of the National Health Service Breast Screening Programme. The cost-benefit of mammography was shown in the trials to be greatest for women aged 50–64 years, partly because of the difficulty in interpreting mammograms from younger women. The essential features of the screening programme are shown below.

The National Breast Screening Programme	
• Method:	Mammography — single oblique views.
• Eligible women:	Aged 50 – 64 years. Women aged over 65 screened on request.
• Frequency of recall:	Every 3 years.
• Organisation:	Regional health authorities have overall responsibility. Screening unit (mobile or static) for a population of approximately ½ million. Assessment centres for follow-up — each covering several screening units.

The role of the practice Although the screening programme is not based in general practice the primary care team has an important role to play by:

1. Promoting uptake
    - Checking prior notification lists issued by FHSA
    - Returning corrected list to FHSA
    - Encouraging attendance
    - Discussing screening with non-attenders.
2. Providing information and counselling
    - Discussing patient's concerns about screening
    - Discussing implications of
        — recall for further investigation
        — biopsy results
    - Discussing treatment options.

The success of the programme in terms of its effect on mortality rates depends both on uptake and the quality of the mammography service and follow-up. General practitioners and their staff have an important role in encouraging patients to attend for screening and providing them with appropriate information and support. This is particularly important for patients who require further investigation in the assessment centres and for those who require biopsy. An estimate of the proportion of women falling into these categories is shown below.

For 2000 patients on a GP's list:

- 150 will be eligible for screening each year
- 7–10 may need further investigation
- 2–3 may require a biopsy
- 1 may have cancer

(After Anstoker 1990)

The main criticism of the breast screening programme has been the low positive predictive value of mammography, which is 5–10%. This means that, out of every 100 positive mammograms, 90–95 will be false positives, causing considerable anxiety for the women concerned. However, there is evidence that improvement in the quality of mammography is resulting in fewer false positives.

DISCUSSION POINTS

Breast cancer screening

Discussing screening procedures with patients may be a searching test of our ability to communicate effectively and sensitively with them.

1. Mrs R, aged 50 years, has just received an invitation to attend the local breast-screening centre. Her sister died recently from breast cancer and she is very anxious and uncertain about having mammography. How would you advise her?
2. Miss T, aged 53 years, has recently had a mammogram and has just received an appointment to attend the assessment centre. She asks you 'What does this mean?'. Outline your reply.

Hypertension

Hypertension is a major risk factor for stroke and, to a lesser extent, for myocardial infarction. Stroke is a significant cause of mortality and disability; in 1989 in England, 100 000 people suffered a first stroke and there were 64 000 deaths from this condition (12% of all deaths). In at least 60% of these hypertension would have been the major risk factor, the risk rising in parallel with rising blood pressure, both systolic and diastolic. There is considerable evidence from a number of studies that reduction of raised blood pressure reduces the risk of stroke. Furthermore, the more effective the reduction in blood pressure towards normal levels, the better the prognosis. The potential benefit from detecting and treating patients with hypertension is therefore great.

What is hypertension? The simple answer is 'raised blood pressure' but this begs the question of the level at which blood pressure is considered to be 'raised'. Blood pressure is a physiological variable which is distributed normally in the population and which increases with age. There is no level at which blood pressure suddenly becomes a risk factor. The risk of stroke increases progressively from the lowest to the highest levels, as shown in Figure 5.7.

Blood pressure varies not only between individuals but also within each individual during the course of the day and is influenced by a number of factors including stress and recent alcohol intake. Thus a diagnosis of hypertension must be based, not on a single reading, but on an average of three readings on different occasions.

For management purposes hypertension is defined as a sustained reading (average of three readings) of 160/95 and above. It can be classified as mild/moderate (95–110 mm diastolic) and severe (over 110 mm diastolic). However, isolated systolic hypertension has been shown to be a significant risk factor for stroke.

Prevention of hypertension Primary and secondary strategies are both important in detecting and preventing hypertension and its sequelae. Development of a *primary* prevention strategy depends on identification of the risk factors for that particular condition. The risk factors for hypertension are:

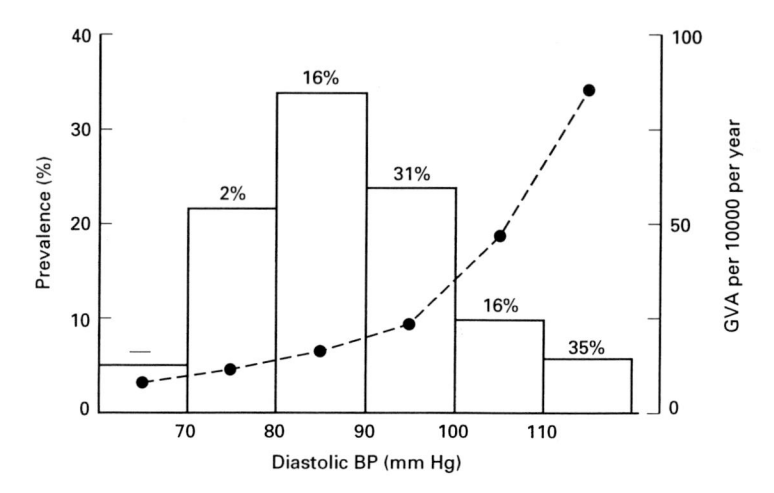

Fig. 5.7 Prevalence distribution (histogram) of diastolic blood pressure related to incidence of stroke (interrupted line). The number above each column is the proportion of all blood-pressure-related strokes arising at that level. Data based on the Framingham Study, men and women aged 35–64 at entry, followed for 16 years. (Published by courtesy of the Royal College of Physicians of London 1989.)

- Family history
- Obesity
- Alcohol consumption
- Salt intake.

Unlike the risk factors for breast cancer, some of those for hypertension are potentially modifiable and primary prevention is therefore feasible. Health education about sensible eating and drinking is clearly important for both the individual and the whole practice population. The association of hypertension with obesity and alcohol consumption above the recommended level is established. For each 14 lb excess in weight, there is an associated 4 mm increase in blood pressure.

Dietary salt intake is also important in the development of hypertension. Recent reports have concluded that salt intake is too high, at twice the recommended level in the United Kingdom and other affluent countries. A moderate reduction in the salt intake of the whole population would lower systolic blood pressure by an average of 5 mm of mercury in those with 'normal' blood pressure and 7 mm of mercury in those with hypertension. This reduction would be expected to reduce the incidence of stroke by about a quarter. This is another example of a *population* prevention strategy. Individuals at *high risk* of developing hypertension and cardiovascular disease should be identified and given appropriate life-style advice.

Screening for hypertension Primary prevention (mainly in the form of advice about life style) and screening must go hand in hand in the detection and prevention of hypertension and its resulting morbidity and mortality. Hypertension is one of the five conditions listed by Mant & Fowler (1990) for which they consider screening to be cost-effective.

DISCUSSION POINT

Screening for hypertension

Look back at Wilson and Jungner's criteria for screening on page 149.
— To what extent does screening for hypertension satisfy these criteria?

Unlike breast cancer, there is no nationally organised programme of screening for hypertension. Although screening may occur in the occupational setting, the onus lies on the general practitioner and the primary health care team who are ideally placed to screen the population and institute and manage treatment of those found to be hypertensive. This is a good example of the desired integration of prevention and care. However, evidence suggests that screening is haphazard. Observations from American surveys led to the formulation of the *rule of halves* which states that half the patients with hypertension are undetected, half of those detected are untreated and half of those treated are uncontrolled. This means that only one in eight of all hypertensive individuals has their blood pressure controlled. Studies have shown that the rule of halves also applies to the detection and management of hypertension in the United Kingdom.

Organisation of screening for hypertension The practice team has a central role in the detection and management of patients with hypertension and, consequently, in the prevention of stroke and, to a lesser extent, myocardial infarction. How is this potential to be achieved? Recent evidence suggests that screening for hypertension in general practice is haphazard, and a structured approach to screening must be adopted to achieve good results.

Screening for hypertension is best achieved by a combination of opportunistic screening or case finding (asking the patient for permission to take a blood pressure when he/she presents in the surgery) and invitations to special screening clinics (e.g. well person clinics). A combination of these two approaches is needed because uptake of invitations to clinics is often disappointing and opportunistic screening will miss the non-consulter.

- The *target population* must be agreed and identified, e.g. everybody in the practice between the ages of 35 and 64.
- *Records* must be kept up-to-date; there should be means of identifying and following up patients who have not had a blood pressure taken and recorded during the past 5 years.
- *A protocol* for the detection and management of patients with hypertension should be drawn up and agreed by all involved in the screening and management of these patients.
- *Training* should be provided for all those involved in screening.
- *Equipment* should be appropriate (e.g. large cuffs), and regularly serviced.
- *Audit* of the detection and management of hypertension should be carried out regularly.

Disease monitoring in practice

Prevention, care and cure should be seen as part of the same continuum, not as separate activities. This is best illustrated by the management of patients with a chronic illness. Monitoring of such patients is an essential part of care, aiming to prevent complications which would lead to death, disability or handicap. This is tertiary prevention.

Care of patients with diabetes and asthma are the best examples of disease monitoring in practice, and clinics held for this purpose attract special payment. Diabetes has been dealt with in an earlier chapter (Ch. 6). The principles of management of patients with diabetes and asthma are similar.

Asthma Asthma is a common condition with an annual mortality of about 2000 in the United Kingdom. The death rate has not changed significantly over the last decade and many of the deaths are preventable. The GP and the primary health care team can play a central role in reducing mortality and improving the quality of life for patients with asthma. The essential features of their role are:

- *Diagnosis*. Remember that asthma often goes undetected and untreated.
- *Prescribing* of appropriate medication.
- Providing *education* and *support* to patients and their relatives.
- *Regular monitoring of*:
  — symptoms
  — patient's concerns
  — lung function (peak expiratory flow rate)
  — inhaler technique
  — medication.

The principles of the organisation of asthma care in practice are similar to those of other chronic conditions, e.g. hypertension and diabetes, and are listed below:

- Identify all patients with asthma in the practice.
- Set up a disease register.
- Develop an agreed protocol for asthma care.
- Decide the structure of care — in asthma clinics or in normal surgeries (not mutually exclusive).
- Identify and train staff involved.
- Obtain and maintain necessary equipment.
- Audit the care you provide.

Prevention of accidents

This chapter will finish by looking at one of the major causes of death and disability, the prevention of which may not figure highly in a practice's list of preventive activities. However, the primary health care team does have an important role to play in accident prevention. One general practitioner commented that he might have achieved more in terms of 'years of life saved' by encouraging parents of young children to fence their garden ponds than all his other prevention efforts.

Accidents are responsible for 2% of all deaths in the United Kingdom and are the biggest cause of death and disability in children, young people and the elderly. Accidents are one of the five key areas identified in the *Health of the Nation* document which sets the target of an overall reduction in accident deaths of 30% by 2005. How is this to be achieved?

Most accidents are potentially preventable, as very few occur by chance. The term 'unintentional injury' is often preferred to 'accident'. In reality, accidents will always occur and the aim must be to reduce not only the overall number but also the risk of death and disability.

Road traffic accidents (RTAs) account for the highest number of deaths of children and young people. The major types of accident for each of the three age groups who are at particular risk are shown below.

Commonest types of accidents in three age groups

Children (1–14 yrs)
- Road traffic accidents (40% of all childhood accidents)
- Drowning
- Poisoning
- Fire
- Suffocation

Young adults (15–35 yrs)
- Road traffic accidents
- Sporting/recreation accidents

Older people (over 65 yrs)
- Falls (responsible for 50% of accidental deaths in this age group)
- Road traffic accidents (20% accidental deaths— mainly pedestrians)
- Fire

DISCUSSION POINT

Prevention of accidents

Select one age group and one type of accident.
— How would you set about reducing the risk of this type of accident for the patients in your practice?

Before considering accident prevention in some detail, there are some important facts to note.

1. There is a marked social class difference in accidental death in childhood. In 1982/3 the SMR for social class I was 80 compared with 180 for social class V. (Remember that the national average = 100.)

2. It is important to be alert to the possibility of *non-accidental* injury in children.

3. *Alcohol* is a significant factor in a large proportion of accidents in young people in particular but also in the elderly.

The ways of preventing accidents can be classified into three groups;

- *Environmental measures*, for example:
  — improving road design
  — designing safe playgrounds.
- *Enforcement measures.* The best example is seat belt legislation which was very effective in increasing the use of seat belts (35% before, to 95% after legislation). This resulted in a 25% reduction in deaths and serious accidents for drivers.
- *Educational measures*, for example:
  — educating cyclists about the value of using helmets
  — educating parents about reducing hazards in the home.

Responsibility for accident prevention lies with many agencies working at different levels in society. These are listed below:

- The individual
- The primary health care team
- Health authorities
- Health education authorities
- Trade unions
- Employers
- Voluntary agencies
- Government departments.

The role of the primary health care team

Health professionals can play a vital role in the prevention of accidents by educational activities.

Educational activities

- General education of patients, e.g. avoiding falls, disposal of unused medicines.
- Education of parents about reducing risks to children in the home, garden, etc.
- Specific advice to those known to be at risk, e.g. on head protection for those taking part in certain sporting activities.
- Enquiry into the causes of individual accidents and advice on prevention of future accidents.
- The hazards of excessive alcohol consumption.

'Medical' activities

- Care in prescribing drugs which may increase accident potential (e.g. psychotropic drugs) particularly in the elderly and those driving or using machinery.
- Diagnosis and management of conditions which may predispose to accidents, e.g. arrhythmias or postural hypotension in the elderly.

Other activities

- Lobbying of local authorities and government about recognised hazards.
- Providing evidence on which legislation can be based, e.g. the reduction in fatal accidents associated with the use of seat belts.

Conclusion

The prevention of accidents is less 'medical' than many of the other disease prevention and health promotion activities we have considered in this chapter. Yet the essential features of an accident prevention strategy are similar to the prevention of specific diseases. These are:

- The whole of the primary health care team should be involved.
- Educational advice should be given to the whole practice population and to specific groups who are at particular risk.
- Health professionals play an essential role in the prevention of disease and the promotion of health but they do so against a backdrop of government legislation, the work of other organisations and the influence of the media.

REFERENCES

Anstoker J 1990 Breast cancer screening and the primary care team. British Medical Journal 300: 1631–1934
Bain J 1990 Child health surveillance. British Medical Journal 300: 1381–1382
Colver A F 1990 Health surveillance of preschool children: four years experience. British Medical Journal 300: 1246–1248
Downie R S, Fyfe C, Tannahill A 1990 Health promotion: models and values. Oxford University Press, Oxford
Fowler G, Mant D 1990 Health checks for adults. British Medical Journal 300: 318–321
Fullard E, Fowler F, Gray J 1987 Facilitating prevention in primary care: a controlled trial of a low technology, low cost approach. British Medical Journal 294: 1080–1082
Grundy R, Dwyer D M 1989 Preventive care card for general practice. Journal of the Royal College of General Practitioners 39: 15–16
Hall D M B 1991 Health for all children: a programme for child health surveillance. Oxford University Press, Oxford
Hart J T 1990 Coronary heart disease prevention in primary care: seven lessons from three decades. Family Practice 7: 288–294
Holland W W, Stewart S 1990 Screening in health care. Nuffield Provincial Trust
Last J M 1963 The iceberg. Completing the clinical picture in general practice. Lancet, 2: 28–31
Mant D, Fowler G 1990 Mass screening: theory and ethics. British Medical Journal 300: 916–918
Marsh G N, Channing D M 1988 Narrowing the health gap between a deprived and endowed community. British Medical Journal 196: 173–176
Morrell D C, Evans M E, Morris R W, Roland M O 1986 The 'five minute' consultation: effect of time constraint on clinical content and patient satisfaction. British Medical Journal 292: 870–873
Royal College of Physicians of London 1989 Stroke: towards better management.
Royal College of Physicians of London 1991 Preventive medicine. A report of a working party of the Royal College of Physicians.
Secretary of State for Health 1992 The health of the nation: a strategy for health in England. HMSO, London

Working Group of the Coronary Prevention Group and the British Heart Foundation 1991 British Medical Journal 303: 748–750

FURTHER READING

Anstoker J, McPherson A 1990 Cervical screening. Practical guide for general practice 14. Oxford Medical Publications, Oxford.
Downie R S, Calman K C 1987 Healthy respect. Ethics in health care. Faber & Faber, London
Jacobson B, Alwyn Smith A, Whitehead M 1991 The nation's health. A strategy for the 1990s. King Edward's Hospital Fund for London, London
McPherson A 1990 Women's problems in general practice. Oxford University Press, Oxford
Priest V, Speller V 1991 Risk factor management manual. Radcliffe Medical Press, Oxford

6. Clinical care in practice

Jeannette Naish, Joe Rosenthal

INTRODUCTION

What do we mean by clinical care? In its broadest sense it might be thought of as everything that goes on between health workers and patients. For the purpose of this chapter, however, we shall use the term clinical care in a narrower way which relates mainly to dealing with people who have 'illness'; although not so narrowly as to consider only those who have 'disease'. We shall think of two broad types of care. The first part of the chapter examines 'episodic care', in which the doctor addresses the problems of patients with acute episodes of illness. Part 2 looks at 'continuing care' or the management of chronic, ongoing problems.

The distinction in reality is often blurred. Acute episodes of ill-health for the patient could vary from short-lived, usually self-limiting common illnesses, to acute exacerbations of a chronic condition and to serious medical emergencies. Patients often use words like 'acute', 'urgent' or 'chronic' in a different way from doctors which is more often related to severity of symptom than duration. The patient may also have different expectations of what can be done for the condition. This difference in understanding and perception of illness often results in the two parties having different agendas when they meet. This could have as much influence as the history, examination and investigation on the management of the problem.

Generally, the doctor is trained to 'cure' disease and the temptation is to intervene by treating, investigating, referring or advising. Patients, on the other hand, may be seeking reassurance or information about how to help themselves. The setting in which episodes of ill-health are presented may also influence management and outcome. For example, the feverish child brought in at the end of evening surgery may well have a very different consultation from one who arrives early in the morning, and the request for an out-of-hours visit to a 'hot' child may be met with telephone advice. The age, sex and personal history of the patient will also affect the way the doctor deals with the problem. An understanding of what influences the patient's decision to consult and their expectations of the outcome is as important as knowledge of the natural history of diseases and of their treatment.

> **Summary of factors that influence clinical management**
>
> - Patient factors
>   — Age
>   — Sex
>   — Race
>   — Symptoms
>   — Expectations
>   — Triggers
> - Doctor factors:
>   — Setting
>   — Perception of patient needs

Part 1
EPISODIC CARE
Jeannette Naish and Joe Rosenthal

INTRODUCTION

This section will deal with the care of illnesses commonly encountered in general practice. Some ideas about factors which influence patients' and doctors' decisions during acute illness will be introduced. These ideas could also apply to other aspects of decision making in general practice. The general principles of episodic care will be outlined and finally, some examples of commonly encountered problems in general practice will be discussed to illustrate some principles of managing episodes of illness, and emergency care in general practice.

WHAT MAKES A PERSON BECOME A PATIENT?

There is a considerable body of research about what happens when people experience symptoms and feel that there is 'something wrong' with their health. Medical help is rarely the first thing that is sought, despite the impression you might have during some surgeries.

People behave in different ways when experiencing symptoms. The term 'symptom iceberg' has been used to describe the fact that not all symptoms lead to a medical consultation, and only one symptom in three is presented to the doctor. More recently, one in eighteen, and one in thirty-six symptoms have been quoted in other studies (Banks et al 1975).

Beliefs and behaviour in illness and health

When a person becomes aware of symptoms suggesting something wrong, family, friends and other members of the lay community are first consulted. Advice and treatment are then recommended. The high street pharmacist may also be consulted for certain problems. Medical help for some people is sought only when the lay referral system fails.

The pattern of lay referral and consultation is influenced by lay beliefs about illness and disease and varies according to different cultures, traditions and ethnic origins (Fitzpatrick et al 1984). That these beliefs are logical and make sense is illustrated by the general practitioner and anthropologist Cecil Helman who proposed a folk classification of illness from patterns of ideas, distinct from medical classifications, about conditions where there were abnormalities in body temperature in a North London community (Helman 1984). For example, when a mother says that she believes her child's diarrhoea is due to teething, her conceptual framework makes perfect sense of this statement, whereas medical teaching would not.

Patients are more likely to agree and comply with the doctor's explanations, recommended treatment and advice if these fit in with their ideas about illness (Tuckett et al 1985). This applies not only to managing illness, but also to health education.

Illness behaviour, or what people do when they feel unwell and seek medical help, is also affected by lay beliefs, cultural influences and traditions (see Ch. 1). A study of how people present their symptoms showed, for example, that the Irish tended to explain their symptoms in somatic terms more than the Italians, who were inclined to be more 'global' and psychologically orientated when describing their symptoms. Thus an Irish person would be more likely to attribute a pain in the head to something wrong with the eyes, ears and so on, whereas an Italian would think about 'nerves'.

There are also 'triggers' which bring people to the doctor. These include perceived interference with vocational, psychological or social functioning, perceived interference with physical activities, or the occurrence of an interpersonal crisis. Sometimes, the decision to go to the doctor is taken by an important 'other person' such as a parent or partner. Another trigger is a sort of time limit the person sets on symptoms, so that if these persist beyond a certain length of time, they are more likely to present them to the doctor.

It has also been shown that an increase in the number of stressful events in individuals' lives makes it more likely that they will notice and present their symptoms to the doctor (Banks et al 1975). This may be true of mothers who bring their children to surgery more frequently than we might think is necessary.

More women than men attend surgery and make use of medical services. Some of their problems are unique but, more importantly, there are differences in perception and expectation between men and women giving rise to different behaviours and attitudes (McPherson 1987).

These are factors that could influence patients' decisions to consult the doctor and the way they present their symptoms. They will also affect patients' perceptions of what the doctor tries to do when formulating diagnoses, treatment and management plans. So it is important that the doctor should not only be aware of them, but also understand how people respond to illness.

DISCUSSION POINT

What makes a person become a patient?

The next convenient time that you see a patient, think about the following questions:
— Why did this person come at this particular time?
— What does this patient believe is wrong?

Summary of factors that influence patients' decision to consult

- Lay beliefs about health and illness influence behaviour.
- There are 'triggers' to consulting the doctor.
- Eliciting the patient's beliefs will help the doctor to formulate a more effective management plan.
- Women and men have different expectations of their health.

CLINICAL DECISION MAKING

A feature of decision making in general practice is related to the aim of separating patients into large binary groups: serious, not serious; urgent, non-urgent; requires a home visit, does not require a home visit; needs laboratory investigations or not, needs hospital referral or not. This distinguishes general practice decision making from that of the hospital specialist who is more concerned with achieving a definitive diagnosis. The general practitioner also sees a much wider range of problems presented at an earlier stage. On the whole, patients in hospital are much sicker than those in general practice. The hospital specialist also has more direct access to laboratory and other investigations, shortening the periods of uncertainty during the diagnostic process.

On the other hand, clinical encounters in general practice extend as a series over time. They are like single frames in a video. These are some of the major differences of content and organisation between general practice and hospital practice. Most of the available research has not demonstrated any significant difference in the thinking processes of generalists and specialists. Both have been described as pattern recognition, hypothesis generating and testing, or probabilistic or predictive. The only difference seems to be that general practitioners ask fewer questions and spend less time on exploring alternative solutions. So the difference is in quantity rather than quality.

Diagnosis is not the only, or the most important, task facing the general practitioner. Choice of treatment and referral are also part of the decision-making process. It is perhaps more relevant to think about this process as one of 'management' of problems presented during encounters with patients, and to remember that decisions have to be taken within the context of the patient's life and culture.

Medical influences on doctors' decisions

John Howie's seminal work on antibiotic prescribing for sore throats illustrated the important influence of the patient's social and psychological history on the doctor's decision to prescribe (Howie 1976 — see p. 196). The doctor's diagnostic uncertainty, a high probability of serious disease and the availability of diagnostic and specialist services are some of the main reasons for referral to the specialist, either for diagnosis, treatment or reassurance.

The question of the appropriateness of referral decisions made by general practitioners has gained prominence since the introduction of the 1990 Contract. A consistent finding is the large variation in referral patterns. However, the samples in these studies are of small numbers of patients referred. For example, one single-handed GP with a list of 2000 may refer less than ten patients to dermatology outpatients, while his neighbour in a group practice of four with 8500 patients may refer 30 or more because he happens to have a special interest in skin diseases.

Some of these findings need cautious interpretation because of the many factors that influence decisions relating to both doctor and the patient. For example, there could be a two-fold difference in consultation rates between practices in the same locality. Allowing that the population characteristics should be similar, and that the list size is not substantially different, what factors could explain this difference in workload? Does a difference in workload or consultation rates explain variations in referral rates? These are all questions needing answers before conclusions about the appropriateness of referral patterns can be drawn.

The influence of clinical epidemiology

It would be fair to say that the phrase 'There is a lot of it about' has an epidemiological basis, although general practitioners may not think of it as such. The next question should be 'Compared with what?'.

Many, if not all, clinical decisions require a knowledge of clinical epidemiology. There was a time when measles and rubella epidemics occurred during alternate years, an item of epidemiological information which was of great help in diagnosing a childhood rash which could be either measles or rubella in appearance.

> **DISCUSSION POINT**
>
> **Clinical decision making**
>
> — What is the evidence to support the statement: 'the cause of your sore throat is likely to be a virus and therefore does not require antibiotics'?

GENERAL PRINCIPLES OF CARE DURING EPISODES OF ILLNESS

Clinical decision making is not simply the process of a patient presenting a problem to a doctor, who then comes to a rational decision for action. Most of the research on medical decision making has been done in hospital practice. McWhinney (1989) proposes a model for general practice which consists of a number of stages in which the doctor systematically goes through the process of formulating 'initial' hypotheses by scanning for clues, then testing the hypotheses before selecting the final hypothesis on which a treatment decision is based.

Howie proposed the hypothesis that therapeutic decisions in general practice do not always follow the route from symptoms, signs, investigations through diagnosis, taking modifying factors into consideration, to treatment. A major alternative route is based on what the patient presents as symptoms straight to treatment decisions which are influenced by the doctor's knowledge of modifying background features such as the patient's social and psychological history. Other important modifying factors include the patient-doctor relationship, and the reasons why people come to the doctor other than for the diagnosis and treatment of illness (Howie 1972).

The availability and accessibility of services also affect what the doctor decides to do. If the local Accident and Emergency unit is more than ten miles away, as it may well be in rural areas, then acute medical problems such as chest pain or diabetic emergencies are dealt with very differently from the inner city with a hospital close by.

In general, 'episodic' care may be about an isolated episode of illness, an exacerbation of a chronic disabling condition, or part of a more prolonged and continuing consultation. The reason why the patient has come is an important part of defining the problem. Then the doctor has to decide whether the problem is or is not urgent/serious/life threatening in medical terms, and whether or not it requires treatment, investigation, referral to a specialist or admission to hospital.

The following are examples of how some symptoms that are commonly encountered in general practice are managed. They are not intended to be about rules, algorithms or recipes of how specific conditions should be dealt with, but more as illustrations of how you might think about the management of specific conditions.

Summary of factors that influence GP decisions

- The consequences of disease for the patient in terms of how the illness affects the performance of her/his normal role.
- The GP's tolerance of clinical uncertainty.
- The patient's social and psychological history.
- The patient's expectations.
- The doctor's knowledge of epidemiological evidence.
- The availability and accessibility of services.

The examples of symptoms used are sore throat, indigestion and back pain. They are chosen because they generally affect different age groups and they vary in duration of symptoms and degree of diagnostic uncertainty. They also differ in the impact they may have on the patient's life.

Sore throat

This example has been chosen because, although it is a very common symptom in general practice with an estimated incidence of 75 cases per 1000 patients per year, there is no standard advice about its management. It raises several questions as to how we manage acute self-limiting illness.

The main source of controversy in dealing with this complaint is when to treat with antibiotics. Bacteria are the causative organisms in less than 30% of sore throats presenting to GPs (Whitfield & Hughes 1981), but earlier studies showed that up to 75% of patients seen were prescribed an antibiotic (Howie et al 1971, Howie & Hutchinson 1978). This percentage has probably since reduced but is still high.

There is no evidence that bacterial infections can be identified clinically (Ross 1971), and a throat swab cannot separate bacterial carrier state from pathological growth. Confirmation of infection requires a rise in the antistreptolysin-0 (ASO) titre, the demonstration of which is not practical in the general practice situation, and it is still not clear if the rapid latex-agglutination test for streptococcal antigen is a sensitive enough tool for use in practice. So how are we deciding when to treat this condition with an antibiotic?

If we consider this problem in the terms discussed above regarding factors that influence doctors' decisions, it seems likely that what probably happens is that we separate patients into two groups: those likely to benefit from antibiotics, and those unlikely to benefit. We allocate to these groups on the basis of a clinical cluster of sore throat, high temperature, enlarged and tender tonsillar lymph nodes and pharyngeal exudate.

Perhaps the most important question is whether we are benefiting those patients for whom we do prescribe antibiotics. Do their symptoms resolve earlier? Are they protected from the potential complications of their possible streptococcal infection? Several studies suggest that the duration of the illness is not much affected by treatment: Whitfield & Hughes (1981) found no reduction in length of illness, irrespective of clinical findings of fever, lymphadenopathy or exudate; Brumfitt & Slater (1957), using parenteral penicillin, found duration shortened by just 24 hours. As for prevention of sequelae, Howie and colleagues, in various studies, showed no reduction in suppurative complications, glomerulonephritis or rheumatic fever.

There is no doubt that another important influence on the decision to prescribe or not is the knowledge of psychosocial factors affecting the patient, for example if they have an imminent examination or major social occasion to attend. Howie (1976) showed the same set of photographs of inflamed throats, but accompanied by different psychosocial background statements, to 634 doctors. It was found that psychosocial factors significantly altered the decision to treat in half the cases.

> **DISCUSSION POINT**
>
> **Sore throat**
>
> — If you had a sore throat and temperature two days before you were due to sit your MRCGP written examination, would you want to take a course of antibiotics?
> — What factors influenced your decision?

We are also influenced by numerous other pressures to put pen to paper (or fingers to keyboard!) and provide a prescription (see box on facing page).

The decision about whether to prescribe for self-limiting illness is not purely academic. Medication of any sort may produce side-effects, is expensive and may reduce patients' confidence in managing such illness themselves. Brooks (1987) describes three 'golden rules' that should be fulfilled in attempting to reduce the number of prescriptions given for such conditions.

Pressures to prescribe
• Urge to 'do something' • Demonstrating concern • Patient pressure and expectation • Fitting with partners' habits • Pressure from pharmaceutical companies • Reducing consultation time • Medico-legal considerations • Possible placebo response • Reducing likelihood of subsequent visit • Playing for time

1. You must really want to stop prescribing for acute self-limiting illness, and for reasons that are in the patient's best interest.

2. Your ideas and intentions must be communicated to your colleagues in the primary health care team, as their behaviour will enhance or diminish your efforts.

3. If you do not offer the patient a prescription then that patient must leave the consulting room believing that he or she has obtained something more valuable.

Summary
• Sore throat occurs in 75 patients per 1000 per year. • Bacteria cause less than 30% of sore throats presenting to GPs. • Bacterial infection cannot be identified clinically. • Duration of sore throat is little affected by antibiotics. • Complications are not reduced by antibiotics. • Psychosocial factors are a major influence on prescribing. • Acute self-limiting illness can be managed sympathetically without writing a prescription.

The purpose of discussing this example has been to illustrate that the management of an apparently straightforward problem in general practice is not a simple matter. The process of deciding on management depends not just on awareness of the currently accepted scientific knowledge but on a complex weighing-up of multiple factors operating in each individual case. You do need to keep up-to-date with developments across the board of clinical medicine but that alone will not make you a 'good doctor'. You must also be aware of the many factors which influence your decision-making and be skilled at discovering your patients' ideas about their problems. In areas of difficulty, do not be afraid of sharing your uncertainty with your patient and negotiating a plan with them.

Indigestion

Indigestion is one of the common complaints which patients bring to the general practitioner. The symptoms tend to recur periodically, with each episode lasting between four and six weeks, with symptom-free intervals. The episodes last longer than sore throats, and do not have the same chronicity as back pain.

What is indigestion?

Patients complain of 'indigestion', while the term 'dyspepsia' is what the doctor usually writes in the records. Prevalence studies show that about 25–30% of a general practice population aged 20 years and over complain of indigestion, and a quarter of them consult their GP (Jones et al 1990). There is a wide variation in consultation rates among GPs in studies of dyspepsia, suggesting that the doctor's style and patients' expectations may influence illness behaviour.

Many definitions for this symptom have been proposed, suggesting that there is a lack of agreement in the scientific world, and indeed, there may be a lack of agreement between the patient and the doctor. While the doctor thinks of 'dyspepsia' as a symptom, 'indigestion' is an already defined condition as far as the patient is concerned, and requires treatment in its own right.

Definitions

In an attempt to clarify the definition of this nebulous condition, an international working party has proposed a classification based on symptoms (Colin-Jones 1988). *Dyspepsia* was defined as upper abdominal or retrosternal pain, discomfort, heartburn, nausea, vomiting, or any other symptom thought to refer to the upper alimentary tract. Symptoms lasting more than four weeks, but unrelated to exercise, and for which no focal lesion or systemic disease could be found were designated *non-ulcer dyspepsia*. *Organic dyspepsia* refers to dyspepsia due to specific disease: peptic ulcer, reflux oesophagitis, carcinoma and so on, identified on routine investigation.

Summary
• There have been many attempts at defining and classifying dyspepsia, suggesting disagreement in the scientific world. • The importance of defining and classifying symptoms of dyspepsia is to differentiate between non-ulcer dyspepsia and serious pathology.

Factors in the aetiology of peptic ulcer

Social class A Medical Research Council special report on occupational factors in the aetiology of gastric and duodenal ulcers in 1951 indicated that social class did not influence the incidence of duodenal ulcers, but that there was a sharp gradient for gastric ulcers, the observed incidence being two thirds less than expected in social classes I and II, and two thirds more than expected in social class V.

Occupation Occupations with a high incidence of peptic ulcer included doctors, business executives and foremen; a significantly low incidence was found among agricultural workers and sedentary workers including civil servants. Workers in the transport industry, skilled and semi-skilled workers showed an average incidence.

Stress and anxiety Related to occupation was the finding that men with duodenal ulcer symptoms complained more often of anxiety about work, but not about home worries. This led to speculation about whether the aetiological factor was anxiety, or a personality type associated with anxiety over work.

Life style and habits Irregularity of meals and shift work were not found to be associated with dyspepsia. But the taking of regular meals is still the routine advice for ulcer sufferers.

The relationship of cigarette smoking, alcohol and coffee consumption has also been studied (Friedman et al 1974). More cigarette smokers than non-smokers reported a history of peptic ulcer. This was the same for both men and women. There did not appear to be a relationship between drinking coffee or alcohol and peptic ulcer.

Infection More recently, in the early 1980s, a strong association between colonisation of gastric mucosa by *Helicobacter pylori* and chronic gastritis has been demonstrated. Many studies have also shown that a majority of patients (70–100%) with duodenal ulcer have gastric *H. pylori* infection. The association with gastric ulceration is also strong. However, the proportion of patients with *H. pylori* gastritis that progress to peptic ulceration is not known.

Treat, investigate or refer?

The difference in decisions about how to manage various common presenting symptoms in general practice depends partly on the degree of

> **Summary**
>
> - There is no clear-cut physical cause for dyspepsia or peptic ulcers.
> - There appears to be a social class gradient in the incidence of gastric ulcers.
> - Occupational factors associated with dyspepsia may relate to stress and anxiety, or to personality types.
> - There is a relationship between cigarette smoking and peptic ulcers.
> - There may be an infective cause for peptic ulcers.

clinical uncertainty that the GP feels. Most people will have tried self-medication by the time they consult their GP about indigestion. The risk of a serious underlying condition, such as carcinoma or peptic ulceration, will influence the choice of options — to treat, investigate or refer. While experience may increase confidence, there will always be clinical uncertainty, be it sore throat, indigestion or back pain. More experienced doctors may tolerate more uncertainty, but there is no need for less experienced doctors to feel inadequate.

Who needs investigation?

Standard medical teaching stresses the need for establishing a firm diagnosis before potent treatments are started for dyspepsia, and it is possible that more referrals for endoscopy and barium meals are made than is necessary. There is ample evidence from studies of abnormal findings from endoscopy or barium meals to demonstrate that younger patients (under the age of 45), with simple dyspepsia, are unlikely to have malignant disorders or any other pathology more serious than simple, non-ulcer dyspepsia. At the same time, older women who regularly take non-steroidal anti-inflammatory drugs are at special risk of peptic ulceration.

Other associated symptoms, such as anorexia, weight loss, vomiting, dysphagia or gastrointestinal haemorrhage, may increase the likelihood of cancer. A failure to respond to simple treatments could also be a warning that there may be underlying malignant disease. The approach to deciding whether or not to investigate should therefore be more clinical than technical, and will have as its basis the knowledge of the clinical epidemiology of dyspepsia.

Endoscopy is the most sensitive investigation for indigestion. A problem arises if endoscopy services are overstretched; there may be less delay for barium studies. In addition, direct access to endoscopy may not be available for general practitioners.

Positive treatment action and choosing what kind

Bearing in mind that most people will have tried self-treatment before consulting the doctor, the decision whether and how to prescribe for indigestion will also depend on the risk of serious underlying disease. The pattern, prevalence, age distribution and associated risk factors of the symptoms of dyspepsia will be the important determinants of the decision to treat and the choice of treatment.

The risk of oesophageal or gastric cancer under the age of 45 is very low and it is now generally accepted that empirical, symptomatic treatment for the younger dyspeptic patient for a short period of time is the correct option. Investigation can be reserved for those who fail to respond to adequate treatment, relapse soon after stopping treatment, or older patients.

Whether simple antacids or the more expensive, ulcer-healing H_2-receptor antagonists are prescribed is a matter of choice. Most symptoms of non-ulcer dyspepsia resolve over 4–6 weeks. There is some logic in choosing simple antacids in the absence of convincing clinical evidence to suggest the presence of peptic ulceration.

Summary

- For young patients (under 45) with dyspepsia, try empirical treatment first, and investigate if they don't respond.
- Patients over 45 with recent onset of dyspepsia, younger patients not responding to treatment and those with symptoms suggestive of cancer need urgent referral for endoscopy.
- Endoscopy is the investigation of choice, but barium studies may be more accessible for general practitioners.

Back pain

Like sore throat and indigestion, back pain is also self-limiting and episodic. But the episodes can be longer, and recur to become chronic back pain. For example, simple muscular back pain can last for four weeks or more. The risk of serious underlying pathology is also less than in indigestion, but the condition is more disabling and distressing for the patient. Everyday activities such as climbing stairs, washing, dressing (particularly putting on shoes and socks), and even shopping or cooking, become much more difficult.

Economically, back pain can result in serious handicap. Recurrent and prolonged episodes can lead to time lost from work and financial loss. It may also mean early retirement from heavy manual work. So back pain can be expensive as well as distressing.

Management

The vast majority of people with back pain do not consult their GP. Over 90% of those who do will recover spontaneously, with the remainder needing referral for investigations. Even some of those who are referred will recover whilst waiting for or undergoing investigation.

Given that there is a low risk of underlying pathology, the decision whether or not to investigate will clearly be more clinical than technical, and be based on the history and examination. For example, one study demonstrated that a history of persistent back pain lasting over one week before presentation, and limited straight-leg raising at the initial examination predicted a poor outcome in terms of recurrence, but not the outcome of the initial episode (Roland et al 1983).

Rather than going through a long list of differential diagnoses, a sensible approach would be to elicit information from the history to decide whether the back pain is mechanical back pain, possible spinal pathology, or nerve root pain (Waddell 1982). Spinal pathology includes infection, inflammatory conditions and tumours which are more common in the older patient.

The degree of distress suffered by the patient may also influence the decision to investigate and treat. The socioeconomic effects of back pain may be so damaging that the patient will search for any solution.

Summary

- History and examination are more important than investigations in diagnostic decisions in back pain.
- The essential differentiation is between mechanical back pain, spinal pathology and nerve root pain.
- Quality of life is an important consideration when deciding how to manage a patient with back pain.
- Patients expect active management because of socioeconomic pressures.

Treating mechanical back pain

It is accepted that, from the day of onset, there is a 90% chance that mechanical back pain will resolve in under 6 weeks. The traditional advice is bed rest and simple analgesia. How much bed rest, which analgesic, and whether anti-inflammatory agents are helpful are open to debate. Most carefully conducted trials of divergent treatments show little or no difference in outcomes. Natural history and the passage of time may be the more effective agents.

Physical treatments include conventional physiotherapy and manipulation. There is a growing body of evidence to suggest that, providing there is no contraindication to manipulation, chiropractic confers long-term benefits when compared with hospital outpatient physiotherapy (Meade et al 1990).

There are other forms of treatment for backache such as acupuncture or massage which can be complementary to the conventional ones, and should be acknowledged. A well-controlled clinical trial of the effectiveness of alternative treatments is awaited. At present, there are many case histories and case series of patients who have benefited, but no clinical evidence to suggest that the effectiveness of these treatments differs significantly from that of conventional methods.

The value of the placebo response should also be recognised. Most treatments and procedures produce a placebo response, unrelated to the established effect of the treatment or procedure, of about 30%, and can last for 3 months.

Summary

- 90% of patients with mechanical back pain recover in under 6 weeks. Natural history and the passage of time may make the most important contribution to resolving mechanical back pain.
- Complementary treatments have a role in the management of mechanical back pain.

Summary of examples

Before going on to deal with emergencies in general practice, what general principles do the above examples illustrate? Although there are similarities between the different kinds of problems that patients bring to GPs, decisions about how to manage each condition are influenced by multiple and complex factors. It would be safe to say that the weighting and combinations of factors are different for each individual case, but general principles do apply.

Defining the problem. This can be thought of as defining the problem from the patient's viewpoint or as defining the medical problem. The two are not mutually exclusive, but understanding patient expectations, patient beliefs, and the effect that symptoms have on people's lives will help in defining the problem in medical terms, and would certainly be helpful in defining the management plan.

The epidemiology and natural history of a condition. It bears repeating that knowledge of the epidemiology and natural history of diseases determines how diagnoses are made and how patients are managed.

The sequelae of episodic illness for patients. In weighing up the pros and cons of treatment, the sequelae of treatment should be part of the equation. Some treatments carry side-effects that may outweigh the benefits. Others are unjustifiably costly in financial terms. The social, psychological and economic impact of the illness may be so severe as to warrant expensive or alternative methods of treatment. It is important to evaluate critically published evidence about investigative procedures and new treatments.

Organisation for service delivery. This applies at practice level as well as outside the practice. As well as patient and doctor factors, effective and efficient organisation allows for better service delivery. The availability of a collection service for pathology specimens may determine whether particular investigations are performed, and referral decisions are clearly influenced by how easy it is to access the particular test or procedure.

EMERGENCIES IN GENERAL PRACTICE

The management of emergencies is a small but important part of general practice. It is impossible to define just what constitutes an emergency and, of course, doctor and patient may have quite different views in particular cases. There is little doubt about certain problems, for example crushing central chest pain or a major bleed, but many presentations are not so clear-cut. Take the example of a child with a rash. This may cause extreme distress for parents until they see a doctor who can reassure them that the cause is a benign one. We can only define what is an emergency in the light of knowledge of the patient's and the family's ideas, culture and experience. We must also take into account the context of the situation. For example, tonsillitis in a teenager may be seen as an emergency if it occurs the week before exams, but not if it occurs the week after.

Differences in perception of what is an emergency can be a cause of stress on several fronts. Typically this may arise with requests for urgent visits, but it may also cause problems for reception staff faced with demands for 'emergency' appointments in the surgery. Different strategies exist for vetting these requests but ultimately we must realise that illness causes great anxiety and that this must be explored even if we feel sure that the problem is unlikely to be a 'true' medical emergency. It is generally wise to see the patient if there is any doubt about the nature of the situation. If a serious condition is not found, then we are in a much better position to educate patients about self-help and appropriate use of services.

One of the aspects of general practice which trainees frequently rate as most stressful is dealing with requests for emergency care out of hours. Assessing situations over the telephone is often a new skill to be developed and this is discussed further in Chapter 4. On many occasions advice over the phone is all that is required or expected. It is wise, however, to state that if the caller is unhappy now or later then you will see the patient. A useful tactic is to specify a period of time after which you will speak to them again, thus giving them a feeling of support and increasing their confidence to deal with the situation with the benefit of your advice. This aspect of the job will get easier with time as your own confidence develops and as you get to know your patients.

In fact the genuine medical emergencies are one thing that medical school and hospital work equip us well to deal with, and we shall not detail the management of specific cases here. You should discuss with your trainer what equipment and drugs you should have available when you are on-call and how to contact ambulance and hospital services. In an emergency situation do not be afraid to call for advice if you need it, either from your trainer or a hospital colleague. Try to remain calm even if all around you are in a state of distress! You will be better able to deal with the task in hand and your confidence will be communicated to the patient and those around you.

Psychiatric emergencies

One type of emergency which frequently engenders a high level of anxiety amongst trainees is the call to a psychiatric emergency. This situation requires tact, understanding and patience. Trainees are often preoccupied with detailed knowledge of the intricacies of the Mental Health Act and procedures involved in compulsory admission. For this reason a brief guide to the Act is given below. A general rule when you decide that a patient requires admission for urgent psychiatric assessment is that you should first aim to persuade them to go voluntarily. Frequently the call for help will come not from the patient but from a relative, friend or neighbour. Try to gather as much information as possible before you visit. Check your notes, look for records of previous problems. If possible, talk to other members of the practice who may know the patient. If there is a history of psychiatric treatment contact the psychiatrist concerned to let them know that a problem may have arisen and discuss the arrangements should you find that admission is required.

A key figure in the management of a psychiatric emergency is the social worker. If you have a strong suspicion that you may need to consider compulsory admission, make early contact to inform them of the situation. Most importantly, you may need to judge whether your safety might be at risk when you visit. If you are worried contact the police. They will accompany you and are skilled at keeping a low profile so as not to aggravate the situation while being on hand should their help be required.

Those trainees who have some experience of hospital psychiatry will naturally be more confident in making a psychiatric assessment but that background is not essential. This is a prime example of a general practice situation where diagnosis is of minor importance relative to making a practical management plan. Your immediate tasks can be summarised as follows:

1. Take a history from the patient and others involved. Where possible try to interview the patient alone in a quiet place.

2. Carry out a physical examination if possible, to exclude an organic problem. This is especially important in elderly patients.

3. Assess the risk of danger to the patient to you and to others.

4. If the problem is one of acute stress, try to discuss tensions and defuse the situation.

5. Decide if it is appropriate to use medication acutely.

6. Decide if admission is essential, and if so whether the patient will go voluntarily.

If you reach a decision that compulsory admission is necessary, the first thing to do is to contact the duty social worker. They will put you in touch with a social worker 'approved' under the terms of the Mental Health Act. They will have detailed knowledge of the Act and can advise on the appropriate Section to be invoked. It is often not realised that the 'application' for most compulsory admissions must be made by the nearest relative or social worker. The doctor's responsibility is not to apply for the order but to make the written medical recommendation. Although the nearest relative can make the application, for practical purposes it is wise to enlist the help of a social worker where possible. One of the reasons for this is that the 'nearest relative' as defined by the Act is not necessarily the person immediately on hand.

Some details of the 1983 Mental Health Act (England and Wales) are given below (HMSO 1983). Note that only patients who cannot be persuaded to enter hospital voluntarily can be admitted under compulsion, and that compulsion should never be used lightly. It is only possible when the patient is suffering from one of the four forms of *mental disorder*, defined by the Act as follows:

1. Mental illness
2. Mental impairment
3. Severe mental impairment
4. Psychopathic disorder.

The Sections of the 1983 Mental Health Act (England and Wales) which are most likely to involve general practitioners are Sections 2, 3 and 4. In Scotland and Northern Ireland different Acts apply.

Section 2

This is a 28-day (maximum, not renewable) order allowing for compulsory admission to hospital of an individual suffering from mental disorder of a nature or degree which warrants detention in hospital for assessment or assessment followed by treatment. Detention must be in the interest of the subject's own health or safety or for the protection of others.

The application must be made by the nearest relative or an approved social worker acting on their behalf. The applicant must have seen the patient within 14 days prior to the date of application. The medical recommendation must be made by two doctors, one of whom must be 'approved' as having special experience in the diagnosis or treatment of mental disorder (usually the consultant psychiatrist or their deputy), and the other who preferably has had previous acquaintance with the patient. Both doctors must have personally examined the patient within 5 days of each other and must state in writing their reasons why compulsory detention is necessary.

Section 3

This is a 6-month (maximum, but renewable) order allowing for compulsory admission to hospital of an individual suffering from mental disorder for the purposes of providing treatment. The grounds for detention are as for Section 2 except that the type of mental disorder must be specified and of a nature or degree which warrants detention in hospital for treatment. The rules as to who must apply and which medical recommendations are required are as follows for Section 2.

Section 4

This is a 72-hour order used to admit a patient to hospital as an emergency and detain him or her for assessment. It only requires one medical recommendation by any registered doctor, as well as an application by the nearest relative or social worker. The grounds for detention are the same as those for Section 2, but it should only be implemented if an undesirable delay would be involved in obtaining the second medical recommendation which is required for Section 2. Both applicant and doctor must have seen the patient within the 24 hours preceding the application.

Completion of the above requirements does not guarantee admission, and acceptance by the hospital must be arranged as well as appropriate transport. Again, the assistance of the police may be required in moving the patient to the hospital.

As you can imagine, the process of sectioning a patient can be very time consuming. If you feel it is safe to do so you can leave the Mental Health Act form with your part completed at the patient's home.

The psychiatric emergency represents a special case of management of emergencies in general practice but a number of general principles are involved.

1. Gather as much information as you can from the initial contact and, where time allows, supplement this with material from notes and colleagues.
2. Always apply calmness and understanding in the emergency situation.
3. History and examination form the basis of management.

4. Diagnosis is often secondary in importance to making a management plan.
5. Knowledge of local resources and specialist skills is essential.
6. Be aware of the limitations to your ability to manage a situation on your own.

Part 2
CONTINUING CARE
Jeannette Naish

INTRODUCTION

The thought of looking after patients with chronic ill-health often evokes negative feelings. Doctors like to 'cure' people and this is not the task required in continuing care. But helping patients and their carers to cope with ongoing illness is as important and just as satisfying a part of the GP's role.

This section will begin by looking at the impact of chronic ill-health upon sufferers and their carers, how it affects the quality of their lives, and how they cope. The ways in which the primary care team and statutory and voluntary services can help to improve the quality of the lives of people needing ongoing care will also be discussed. Finally, some examples of chronic disabling conditions will be examined in order to illustrate some general principles of continuing care.

The cornerstones of general practice are primary, personal and continuing care. The clinical aspects of care are a significant part of the story, but by no means the whole. There are many general issues involved in caring for people, some of which are essential parts in the everyday life of a general practitioner. These areas will also be addressed.

THE IMPACT OF CHRONIC DISEASE

The experience of recurring, distressing symptoms is a feature of some, but not all chronic diseases. For example, patients suffering with arthritis will experience pain, while a patient with hypertension may have no symptoms.

The World Health Organization proposes a model for determining the degree of disability resulting from chronic disease.

Impairment refers to the organic disease, where there is abnormal physiological, physical or psychological function. This may or may not lead to *disability*. For example, the loss of a little finger on the left hand of a right-handed labourer will cause little disability, but will be disastrous for a violinist. Whether disability creates a *handicap* will depend on how the individual copes with the disability, what resources are available to help, and the coping strategies that are adopted.

Sometimes, impairment can lead directly to handicap by virtue of its 'stigmatising' potential: in the sense that it marks the sufferer as being different, and inferior in some way. Some medical conditions are stigmatising without causing any obvious disability, giving rise to social and vocational disadvantages.

Epilepsy is a condition which may not be associated with any significant disability, but could lead to handicap because of the potential to stigmatise. In their report of interviews with 94 adult epileptics, Scambler & Hopkins (1986) found that patients felt alarmed and despondent when they were told that they were suffering from epilepsy. The image of 'epileptic' carried the likelihood of being discriminated against and of being inferior. Practical consequences such as long-term medication, not being allowed to drive, and decreased career opportunities were foremost in people's minds.

It is important that the doctor does not only think about the management of chronic disability in medical terms, but also in terms of the social and psychological consequences of chronic illness for the patient and carers. These will depend on how disabling the condition is, and whether or not it leads to handicap. How much help is needed for the patient to cope will be determined by the patient's personal resources (in both the psychological and economic sense), the presence of lay carers to give social and practical support, and the availability and quality of statutory and informal services.

Personal resources

As we have said, some conditions are potentially stigmatising. Psychiatric illness is an example of how social disadvantage is acquired through being labelled as mentally ill, and is never lost even if the patient recovers. At the same time, the patient's perception of stigma may be worse than the actual experience of discrimination, as Scambler & Hopkins found in their study of epileptic adults (1986). The perception that one is abnormal and different is the primary source of stigma.

Coping with chronic illness

Considerable effort is needed for the patient to adjust to and cope with this sense of stigma. Various 'coping strategies' have been described. Some patients adjust their expectations to accommodate their illness, actively taking an interest in their condition and generally having a positive attitude. Some try to find compensation and benefits in being chronically ill, enjoying dependency or social withdrawal. A third way of coping is to deny and minimise the condition, attempting to live as though the illness did not exist. Another is to resign oneself to the condition, being passive and hopeless, and letting the illness dominate everything.

Sometimes, the coping strategy that is adopted may miss the point and may therefore be inappropriate, the 'heart sink' patient being a special example. Whatever advice the doctor gives is never enough to help solve the problem. The individual then may need help either from her/his social network or the medical profession.

Economic disadvantage

Career advancement and employment prospects may well be affected by chronic illness, resulting in reduced income. The disabled are more likely to be unemployed, and if in employment, likely to earn less than the non-disabled, with the most severely disabled earning the least.

Whilst there are state benefits to supplement and support disabled people living in the community, the general practitioner, as the agent of society, is often required to adjudicate on the validity of a patient's claim for benefits. The administrative criteria for claiming benefits are usually rigid and dichotomous, applied with certainty and at a point in time. The doctor is more often uncertain, with diagnoses being provisional and to be negotiated with the patient.

For example, patients are often not told that they may have multiple sclerosis (MS) after the first or second episode of demyelination. This is usually because intervals between exacerbations could be long or short, and the diagnosis could be in doubt. As MS is a serious and potentially disabling condition, the wish to ameliorate bad news and a genuine uncertainty about prognosis could lead the doctor to 'wait and see'. This is to avoid worrying the patient unnecessarily, which could lead to serious harm; the patient may become severely depressed or suicidal on being given a serious diagnosis. Thus, the diagnostic uncertainty of the doctor delays the application of a disease label, with the result that the patient cannot claim benefits.

The advantages and disadvantages of telling a patient about the diagnosis of a disabling illness have to be carefully balanced. General practitioners can be very helpful in encouraging their chronically sick patients to claim benefits and allowances by informing them of their entitlements (Table 6.1), and explaining the complexities of claiming.

The carers

The quality and availability of social and practical support are important influences on how well chronically sick people cope with their disabilities. The major burden of care lies with relatives and family members, who are often female. Statutory and informal community services to support the disabled living at home vary between districts, and generally serve to supplement the care given by relatives, close friends and neighbours, often coming into operation when the lay carer breaks down. Not surprisingly, many carers experience considerable psychological distress.

The general practitioner and other members of the primary care team concerned with caring for chronically ill and disabled patients need to monitor the wellbeing of carers as well as their patients. A break from the unremitting daily chores of looking after an elderly, confused relative or

Table 6.1 Social security benefits

Finance	Apply to:
Invalidity pension and allowance (after 28 weeks sickness benefit)	Local Social Security Office
Industrial disablement benefit — is result of work-related injury or disease	Local Social Security Office
Severe disablement allowance — people of working age who do not quality for national insurance benefits	Local Social Security Office
Attendance allowance — need attention in connection with bodily function: supervision to avoid substantial danger to himself or others. High rate — day *and* night Low rate — day *or* night	Address on leaflet
Invalid care allowance — people of working age looking after disabled relative on Attendance allowance.	Address on leaflet
Income support — qualification depends on income, personal allowance and premiums according to circumstances (age, disability, family carers, single parent)	Local Social Security Office
Social fund for people on Income support- Community care *grants* — one-off payments for elderly, frail people with disabilities, families under stress. Social fund *loans* for people in particular need—repayable, no interest charge	Local Social Security Office
Housing benefit — rent/community charge	Local Authority Housing or Finance Departments
Independent living fund — regular payment for purchase of care — aged 16–74 — on higher rate attendance allowance — in need of personal and domestic care — discretionary	Address on form

Note: Disability Organisations/Advice Centres in many areas provide advice on any of the above. Rules and regulations change, so this list may be out of date. It is worth checking up from time to time.

spouse may make all the difference to the mental health of a carer. Local facilities vary and may be restricted, but as well as provision for helping with personal care, there are usually facilities for day care, respite care and sometimes the voluntary services of someone who would sit with the patient while the carer goes out.

THE ROLE OF THE GENERAL PRACTITIONER IN CONTINUING CARE

The care of people with chronic illness requires integration of the many different skills of general practice. Since the 1990 Contract, there has been a risk of general practice becoming compartmentalised into 'mini' clinics of various types. This approach may work for certain well-defined problems but in many chronic illnesses it does not succeed.

Medical care

The medical part of continuing care concerns monitoring the effects of treatment, how the patient is progressing and, most importantly, the early diagnosis and prevention of the complications of disease (tertiary prevention). This involves regular review and a systematic examination of patients on long-term medication. The use of clinical protocols is often advocated. The process of writing a protocol should allow the doctor(s) to consider what constitutes good clinical practice in the management of a particular chronic condition.

It is important to ensure that patients comply with advice about taking medication and adopting more appropriate life styles. This requires the doctor to give comprehensive and comprehensible information as well as being perceptive to the patient's beliefs and concerns. The issues to communication are dealt with in more detail in Chapter 4.

Social support

The importance of social support in promoting better coping strategies for people living with disability has already been mentioned. Empathy, compassion and continuity are important to patients and carers. Seeing a patient regularly, especially when it requires a home visit, may not seem to be an efficient use of time in the medical sense, but could mean a lot to the patient and carers as an expression of interest and concern and provide a source of emotional support.

Time constraints mean that most GPs have to be selective about visiting chronically ill people at home. This is another item on a long list of ethical dilemmas facing the GP every day — one of deciding about priorities. In general, a person with good social support would be less likely to be on the chronic visiting list than isolated older people living alone.

Most, if not all, general practitioners give supportive psychotherapy, sometimes without knowing. Michael Balint (1957) was the first to describe this phenomenon. If the role of the GP as a generalist is to be persevered, then this supportive role must remain.

EXAMPLES OF CONTINUING CARE IN THE COMMUNITY

Community care is mostly about supporting and enabling people with chronic disabilities to lead as full a life as possible with a maximum degree of independence, in the community. The priority groups are people with mental illness or mental handicap, the elderly, and those with a physical or sensory handicap. The first three are the focus of the Community Care Act due to become operational in 1993, when local authority social service departments will assume overall responsibility for providing community care.

A range of services is required to meet the needs of people with chronic disabilities, provided by a variety of agencies including statutory health and social services, and informal, voluntary agencies. A multidisciplinary team approach to planning and delivering services is essential at most if not all levels of service provision. Where aims and goals are shared, good communication and cooperation are important for effective collaboration. Services are often limited, and good teamwork is one way of sharing and maximising the efficient use of scarce resources.

The following are some examples of care in the community, focusing primarily on general practice. They are not intended to be a comprehensive list of examples, but to illustrate the general principles of continuing care.

Community care of people with a mental handicap

Many people find the label of 'mental handicap' offensive and degrading. Through the years, many different names have been tried and discarded: mentally defective, retarded, ineducable, educationally subnormal, idiot, and so on. 'People with special needs' has been a popular label, but can also refer to people with sensory or physical handicaps. Throughout this chapter, the term 'mental handicap' will be used.

What is mental handicap?

Mental handicap has been defined as a 30% or greater deficit in developmental and cognitive skills leading to intellectual retardation, social incompetence and educational backwardness. The prevalence of profound and severe handicap, defined as an IQ of less than 50, is roughly 3–4 per 1000 population; between 6 and 8 patients in an average general practice list of 2000. Mild handicap, defined as IQ 50–70, may be ten times greater. The relationship that the general practitioner has with mentally handicapped people and their families can last a lifetime. Although the prevalence of mental handicap in general practice is low, its management illustrates the benefits of a multidisciplinary approach where services are provided by statutory health, education and social services, and voluntary agencies.

Historical note

The public at large hold negative images of people with a mental handicap. This is probably because of difficulty in coping with intellectual and physical disabilities, unacceptable behaviours and fear of hereditary implications, often based on hearsay and folklore.

The traditional forms of care for mentally handicapped people arise from ignorance of the nature of the disabilities and handicaps. Large institutions were built in the late nineteenth and early twentieth centuries, designed to care for people who could not be looked after by their families or local communities. They were set well away from busy centres of social and commercial activity, but at the same time provided peace and quiet, often in pleasant rural surroundings. Patients were safe but out of sight.

Community care

With increasing knowledge of the nature of handicap, and the development of new treatment methods, the traditional way of managing mentally handicapped people is no longer acceptable, although services for helping people with a mental handicap to live in the community are not always adequate. Since the early 1950s there has been a growing belief that many of the physical, psychological and behavioural problems associated with mental handicap could be best managed in the community.

Along with the elderly, mentally ill and chronically disabled who had previously been cared for in long-stay institutions, mentally handicapped people are being integrated into society. Health and local authorities are transferring people from the large gothic institutions to small community homes and hostels, local specialist units and their own homes. Primary care services will provide for some of their needs, and general practitioners are expected to provide general medical services.

Because of the tradition of caring for mentally handicapped people in isolated institutions, and the low prevalence of severe mental handicap, family doctors have had little experience of the problems particular to this group of people and their families. Learning opportunities during both undergraduate and postgraduate training are few. So the average GP is poorly prepared to assume responsibility for a small, but significant and increasing, number of patients with special needs.

Medical needs

Mentally handicapped people suffer with coughs, colds, aches and pains and anxiety and depression just like everyone else, but their medical needs may be greater. A prospective study comparing the care of 134 children with Down's Syndrome with 134 controls, matched for age and sex, aged between 1 and 10 years and living with both parents in Scotland in 1981 found that the Down's children were twice as likely to have contact with their GP, with a three-fold increase in the number of home visits (Murdoch 1984). They were twice as likely to be referred to the paediatrician, and twice as likely to be admitted to hospital. The majority of problems were respiratory.

There are other conditions to remember when seeing someone with Down's Syndrome. For instance, there is a higher prevalence of hypothyroidism among people with Down's, so it is worthwhile screening thyroid function from time to time. Children with Down's Syndrome are more likely to have hearing impairment from glue ear, which is particularly difficult to treat. Congenital heart disease and visual impairment are also more common. The GP also has a role in monitoring the side-effects of drugs and treating intercurrent illness.

The GP's major contribution stems from knowledge of the social and psychological history of the families and carers. Anxieties and misconceptions about medical conditions are potentially disabling. The family doctor can do much to support these people in helping them to work out their coping strategies.

Physical and sensory impairment

People with severe mental handicap are often multiply handicapped. Associated neurological abnormalities lead to gross and fine motor disabilities. There are also problems with proprioception, resulting in abnormal coordination and balance, and ataxia. This affects mobility and aspects of self-care such as dressing and feeding. Modern physiotherapy methods, often linked with behaviour modification techniques, can sometimes help to improve muscle control and movement, limiting the disabilities to some extent. Aids to daily living, housing adaptations, walking aids and wheelchairs may also be necessary.

Visual and hearing impairment can sometimes go undetected in people with mental handicap, due partly to the difficulties of assessment. Sadly, this can make learning difficulties worse than they need be.

Services and resources

Resources for helping people with multiple handicaps are provided by either the local authority social service department or health service community mental handicap services. The Department of Health will provide wheelchairs and other aids to mobility. Generally, social services will provide the aids and adaptations to the home, and are responsible for residential and day care. Social workers will also do case work, support the families and carers, counsel when needed, coordinate services and facilitate access to services.

The health service provides the specialist, professional carers such as physiotherapists, community mental handicap nurses, occupational therapists and psychiatric services, in the form of the Community Mental Handicap Team. Members of the team will perform the assessments and also plan and provide treatment. Other members of the primary care team will be involved from time to time.

Voluntary bodies — such as MENCAP, the Spastic Society, Down's Syndrome Society, and the Rowantree Trust — will often provide help such as equipment grants or holidays.

Social security benefits and allowances are often of primary importance, with the Disability Living Allowance being the most helpful. Welfare benefits are changing all the time, and it is important to keep up-to-date.

Clearly, with so many agencies involved, joint planning of services is essential in caring for these groups of people.

Children with mental handicap

Some children with mental handicap are identified by the paediatrician or GP in the neonatal period. More commonly, learning difficulties emerge over the first few years of life. The recognition of developmental delay is one of the main reasons for having a child health surveillance programme.

Some causes of mental handicap

The causes of mild mental handicap are, in most cases, unidentified. The basis of severe mental handicap is more likely to be known but may also be obscure. However, explanations are helpful for parents and carers who may find it easier to accept the handicap if they can understand the reasons for it. At the same time, knowing some of the causes for mental handicap will help the general practitioner to think about prevention and counselling for subsequent pregnancies.

Preventing handicap

Ensuring that all women embarking on their first pregnancy are immune to rubella is something that is feasible in general practice. Similarly, encouraging diabetic mothers-to-be to achieve good control, smokers to stop smoking, and talking to patients about screening for chromosome and other fetal abnormalities are all within the scope of general practice antenatal care.

The debate about the costs and benefits of childhood immunisation is more complex, but concerns all parents. A significant proportion of severe brain damage is the result of head injuries, whether accidental or not, so the prevention of accidents and being alert to non-accidental injuries to children is of concern to general practitioners.

Similarly, the GP should be on the lookout for early signs of hypothyroidism, diabetes and other conditions that may contribute to mental handicap.

The psychology of mental handicap

It has been said that a family with a handicapped child is a handicapped family which is at risk of social isolation: isolation from the extended family, marriage under strain, maladjusted siblings and crises or breakdown. The emotional responses to the realisation that a child is imperfect are like the bereavement response, but much modified.

There is mourning for the perfect child, but unlike in death, the imperfect child remains. There is extra work in caring for a handicapped child, disturbed nights, and recurring disappointments at the failure to attain expected milestones.

Emotional adjustment

Parents and family members of a handicapped child work through the stages of bereavement at different rates.

The parents often differ in this process because of the mother's closer contact with the child. Often, helping agencies concentrate more on the mother's emotional needs, leaving father to fend for himself. He is also often at work when the health visitor or social worker calls during the normal working day. Siblings may develop disturbed behaviour, with teenagers having a particularly hard time, having to cope with the arrival of a handicapped sister or brother as well as their own growing up.

Not surprisingly, maladaptive responses to the bereavement process can occur. The general practitioner has an important role in monitoring this process, and understanding some of the parents' demands which may at first seem unreasonable.

The GP can help at various stages; she or he needs skills, in particular in breaking bad news and in helping the family to cope with living with a handicapped child.

The caring professions are there to help families cope through the bereavement process, prevent isolation, learn to care for the handicapped child and help the child to realise her/his potential.

Coping with difficult behaviours

Behaviour modification techniques are often employed to help overcome socially less acceptable behaviours such as incontinence, poor independent living skills such as feeding and dressing, temper tantrums and attention-seeking behaviour. This method is based on the principle of immediate reward for the desired behaviour; anyone familiar with potty training will

Breaking bad news

Three critical times:

- *Birth.* There may be obvious congenital abnormalities. This is the arrival of the imperfect baby.
- *Development.* Handicaps become apparent as the child develops. The commonest time is when the child is aged 2–3 years, when learning difficulties appear.
- *Following illness or accident.* Parents had been facing the prospect of the child's death, sometimes preferring death. The perfect child becomes imperfect and a different child has to be taken home.

How the family doctor can help families to cope with living with a handicapped member

- Help and support during the bereavement process. Facilitate contact with other members of the primary care team and other professional agencies (e.g. MENCAP, Spastic Society).
- Help and facilitate contact with other families with a handicapped child, e.g. local parents' groups.
- Help the child to reach maximal developmental potential. This may involve knowledge of special services and facilities. The local mental handicap team and community paediatrician are good sources of information.
- Help to support parents through difficult behaviours such as tantrums, incontinence, and so on.
- Provide practical help and information about aids and equipment, welfare benefits, voluntary organisations, transport, and so on.
- Look after the medical needs of the child and the emotional wellbeing of the parents and carers.

have come across this. The difficulty is in dealing with a handicapped child who takes longer to learn, and each task has to be broken down into much smaller steps to be taught and learned in a logical sequence. The principles of behaviour modification also apply to helping handicapped adults to learn new skills or to improve existing ones.

Residential care

There may come a time when parents and families are no longer able to care for a mentally handicapped person at home, through ill-health, disabilities and so on. Local authorities provide residential care to varying degrees, catering for a variety of abilities. Some function as hostels, others are small group homes where the residents manage with some degree of supervision. Private homes are also available, and some voluntary organisations, such as the Spastic Society and Home Farm Trust, have special provision for particular needs. Short-term respite care is often much needed and most residential establishments have provision for respite care.

A special group are people with so-called challenging behaviours. These are extremely aggressive or violent behaviours, and intractable self-injuring behaviours. Medication and behaviour modification programmes sometimes help, but custodial care in special units may be the only solution when family and community services cannot cope.

Day care

Most children with mild mental handicap are now integrated into mainstream schools. 'Special' schools are available for the more profoundly handicapped, particularly if there are associated physical and sensory handicaps.

In theory, it should be possible for the person with mild mental handicap to obtain employment on the open market to perform simple tasks. Local and health authorities also provide day-care facilities for adults, although this varies from no provision, particularly for profoundly handicapped adults, to active Adult Training Centres where vocational and educational activities take place. Leisure activities are also catered for in some areas, in the form of social clubs, parents' groups and so on.

In most areas the social service departments are responsible for finding suitable day and residential facilities when needed.

What lessons can we learn from caring for people with a mental handicap in the community?

- *Prevention.* The GP has an important role in preventing mental handicap.
- *Team work.* Community care for people with a mental handicap requires well-organised multidisciplinary teamwork.
- *Coordination.* The GP has a role in coordinating service delivery for people with mental handicap.
- *General medical services.* The GP has a challenging role in the general medical care of people with mental handicap.

Health care for older people

The proportion of the UK population over 75 is rising dramatically and this is reflected in the work of GPs in most areas. On the whole, older people are those who have survived and coped, and they are generally healthy. So it would be quite wrong to think that they have special needs simply because of age. However, the aims of health care for the elderly are different in some ways. In 1990 the Royal College of General Practitioners published an occasional paper *Care of Old People* (Baker 1990), which offers a useful framework for looking after older people in general practice.

Objectives of GP care of older people
1. To maintain and, where possible, improve the quality of life for elderly people by a regular programme of medical audit.
2. To keep abreast of new developments in health care by a commitment to continuing medical education.
3. To take into account old people's problems in gaining access to the available services provided by the practice.
4. To strive to reach accurate diagnoses on which logical treatment and realistic progress can be based.
5. To provide effective continuing care for those with long-term medical problems and chronic illness.
6. To offer a systematic programme of anticipatory health care for older people.
7. To contribute to the resettlement of patients who are discharged from hospital or other institutions back into the community.
8. To provide sensitive and effective care for the dying patient.
9. To develop and participate in a team approach to the provision of the care of elderly persons.
10. To provide information and health education to older people in the practice.
11. To support the informal carers with the aim of preventing breakdown.
12. To further the interests of older people and, when necessary, act as their advocate.

What happens in practice

General practitioners will plan care for their elderly population depending on local needs and resources. Teamwork is essential to delivering a good service to older people.

The main aim of health care for older people is to help them to maintain independent living in the place of their choice. Most people like to live in their own homes, and with support may choose to continue to do so in spite of enormous difficulty. The question of moving is in many cases first raised not by the old person but by their family or neighbours. This may cause considerable distress for someone who has to leave the home where they have lived for many years, brought up a family, and which often holds memories of a deceased spouse. Informal carers can also be reluctant to 'put Mum/Dad away' into an old people's home. The general practitioner who knows the patient and the carers well can perform a major part in supporting people through the decisions which have to be made during difficult times.

The patient's view

Elderly people often say that they are in 'good health' despite having one or more medical conditions requiring medication. This usually depends on

> **DISCUSSION POINTS**
>
> **General practice issues in healthcare for older people**
>
> — What are the ethical dilemmas when deciding where an old person should live if their current housing is unsuitable?
>
> — What are the ethical dilemmas when deciding whether a confused old person should be admitted into institutional care?
>
> — Should the issues of terminal care be discussed before a person becomes terminally ill?
>
> — When resources are scarce, what are the ethical dilemmas relating to the allocation of community services for people who are highly dependent, but living in the community?

how much the condition interferes with daily living or leisure activities. For example, someone suffering with hypothyroidism, but well controlled on replacement therapy, should have little difficulty in coping with the demands of normal daily living, whereas a stroke victim left with some degree of hemiparesis would be handicapped by impairment of motor function and would require support services: a home help for coping with domestic duties, the district nurse for aspects of personal care, the chiropodist to help look after feet, help with transport, and possibly day care or respite care to relieve informal carers may all be needed. So the concepts of impairment, disability and handicap are again relevant when thinking about health care for older people. Teamwork and good communication between the agencies involved, including practice staff such as receptionists and practice nurses, are more important than ever.

Regular review of medication

Another important aspect of caring for older people is the regular review of medication. People over the age of 65 are more likely to be taking medicines than those younger, and are also likely to be taking more than one medicine. Apart from practical problems due to poor vision, poor memory or impaired dexterity, poor hepatic and renal function can lead to drug toxicity. We must be on guard for side-effects and interactions. A study of repeat prescribing of non-steroidal anti-inflammatory drugs in Northern Ireland found that over a quarter of patients taking these agents were also on anti-hypertensive treatment, when hypertension can be iatrogenically caused by NSAIDs (Steele et al 1987).

Medical education and hospital practice tend to emphasise the 'medical model' of diagnosis, investigation and surgical or medical treatment. The idea of maintaining quality of life is perhaps given more priority in general practice where we see people in their own surroundings. The social and supportive role of the doctor and the value of a relationship built up over many years are illustrated by the following case history.

> **DISCUSSION POINTS**
>
> **Medication for older people**
>
> — Are some of your elderly patients prescribed codeine-based analgesics and laxatives at the same time?
> — If so, is this logical?

Queenie was born in 1876 and died at the age of 102. I first met her when she was a hale 84-year-old with ischaemic heart disease and chronic bronchitis. She was taking 10 different tablets every day, and came to see me in our geriatric surgery once every two months to get her tablets and have her heart, chest and blood pressure checked. We were fortunate in having a weekly geriatric ambulance provided by social services for those patients who had difficulty in getting to the surgery. She was living with her married daughter May, and May's husband and son. The grandson married when Queenie was 95, but continued to live with May, so that when the baby came along two years later, there were four generations living together in a three-bedroomed council house. By then, Queenie was confined to the ground-floor living room, being unable to walk more than a few yards without chest pain and unable to climb stairs. A bed had been made up for her there. I was visiting her about every six to eight weeks to give her a prescription and check her heart, chest and blood pressure. We celebrated Queenie's century in the surgery. She came to the party in an ambulance.

Somehow, the medical routines became of secondary importance despite the fact that Queenie regularly had her renal and liver function and her digoxin levels checked. While these routines were being performed, there were interesting and quite often prolonged discussions about the baby, the family in general and, more importantly, how May was coping with Queenie's increasing dependence. In fact, she coped beautifully, but at considerable emotional cost and, unknown to Queenie, was also coming to see me in surgery with bouts of anxiety and depression. Yet in spite of everything, May would not countenance hospital admission when Queenie's foot became gangrenous. She nursed her to the last, declining all but the minimum help from the District Nurse. I like to think that my regular home visits helped May to achieve this.

Queenie's story is not unique, nor does it describe all the areas relating to the care of older people. The main issues are that the follow-up arrangements depended on access, that transport was available to bring Queenie in to surgery when she was able to come, and later she was visited at home when she became confined to one room. She was very well cared for by her daughter who needed some help from time to time, but, except at the end, nursing and other community services were not required. Her medical condition was regularly reviewed. But this is not the whole story.

Some of it can only be learned through the experience of caring for people such as Queenie.

Summary

- A care plan for a dependent, older person living at home will be determined by the needs of that person and the availability of local resources.
- Informal carers have the major burden of community care.

Preventive care of older people

The 1990 Contract makes specific proposals for care of the elderly. Doctors are now required to offer annual visits to their patients aged 75 years and over and to carry out a comprehensive surveillance programme. Recognition of the increase in workload that this entails is reflected in the substantial increase in capitation fees for patients in this age group. The Contract does not specify that the doctors themselves must carry out the programme, and other members of the team are often involved.

The over-75-year checks required by the NHS

GPs should offer all their patients aged 75 and over an annual home visit to perform a review in the following areas:

- Sensory functions
- Mobility
- Mental condition
- Physical condition, including continence
- Social environment
- Use of medicines.

A review of the studies published so far shows that there are few clear benefits from screening the elderly, while the implications for the increase in workload could be daunting. It is agreed that there are unreported needs amongst the elderly population, but follow-up studies raise questions about the effectiveness of screening this group.

Taylor & Buckley (1987) reviewed developments in preventive care of the elderly. A number of case finding/screening programmes were described and evaluated. The team approach, with health visitors or nurses taking the lead, appears to be an effective way of operating a screening programme for older people. Screening by postal questionnaire was also useful in detecting common problems. The idea of targeting high-risk groups for more intensive surveillance is an attractive one. The concept of 'risk' relates to the impairment of social, psychological and physical functioning rather than susceptibility to disease. This could well be the most important reason why clear benefits from screening the elderly have not been demonstrated if the expected outcomes are about improvement in medical conditions. Thus, a systematic functional assessment becomes the major focus of screening. However, doctors are not formally trained to do systematic functional assessment, although illness will affect function at all levels.

Williams (1986) proposes a scheme for thinking about the ability to perform activities of daily living at three levels: relating to the outside world, performing domestic tasks, and personal care. These relate to each other dynamically, which is illustrated by putting each level as a series of concentric rings around the person (Fig. 6.1). All the rings have to be intact for fully independent living.

Summary

- The ideas of tertiary prevention are central to caring for older people.
- The main aim of care of the elderly is not of 'cure' or improvement in the disease, but the alleviation of suffering and maintenance or improvement of the levels of functioning and quality of life.

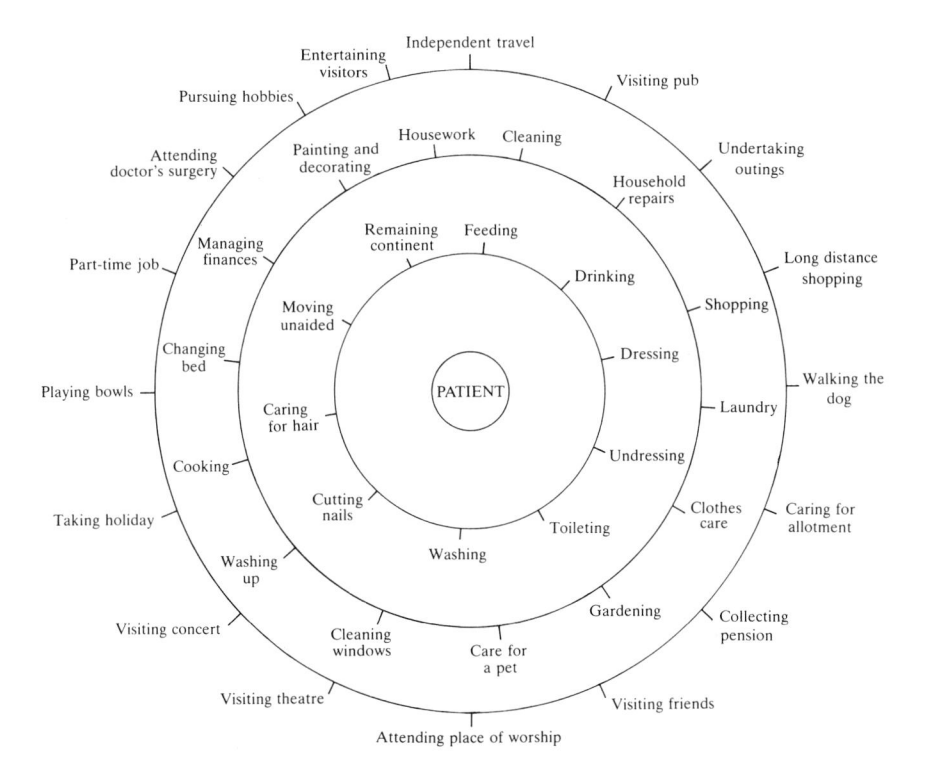

Fig. 6.1 Social performance levels of elderly persons. (From Williams 1986. Reproduced with permission of the Editor of the *British Journal of General Practice*.)

- Established disease needs to be recognised early, whether during chronic disease monitoring or active screening.
- Social support or treatment should be initiated to minimise possible functional impairment caused by illness, and to improve the quality of life.

Psychiatry in general practice

What do we mean by psychiatry in general practice? Do we mean the care of people with chronic mental illness? Do we mean minor psychiatric disturbances, notably anxiety and depression? Or do we mean the care of people who feel miserable and unable to cope with the complexities of modern living?

The specialty of psychiatry is mostly concerned with the study of abnormal human behaviour. It is impossible to define what constitutes 'normal' behaviour and so mental illness has no straightforward diagnostic criteria. Once again, the social context of the patient's life and the person's coping strategies will determine whether emotional disturbances are presented to the GP and what, if any, form of intervention is needed. The experience and interest of the GP will influence the detection rate. When faced with a patient who has emotional or behavioural problems, the GP is not so much concerned with diagnosis as answering questions such as the following:

- Is this a social or a psychiatric problem?
- Is intervention needed?
- Should medication be prescribed?
- Would counselling help?
- Can I help this patient on my own?
- Could other members of the team help?
- Should a referral be made to a hospital?
- What is the natural history of this condition?
- How can I prevent this problem recurring or getting worse?

The nature of psychiatric problems in general practice

Morbidity statistics from the RCGP Second National Study (1971–72) suggest that more than half of psychiatric consultations are for psychoneuroses. About a third of these are somatic disorders of psychological origin, such as tension headache and insomnia. The psychoses, dementias, mental retardation, personality disorders and alcohol or drug abuse together contribute one-sixth of consultations for psychiatric disorder. Hospital admissions show the opposite trend, where psychoneuroses account for one-tenth of all admissions, with the bulk taken up with the psychoses, mental retardation and dementia.

The trainee who has worked as a psychiatry SHO will have had considerable experience of hospital psychiatric problems but less of the 'minor' psychological problems which are so common in general practice.

Minor psychiatric disorders This is a term loosely used to cover problems such as depression, anxiety and somatic complaints of psychological origin. Although they are described as minor they are very often chronic and need continuing care. The limitations of classifications in general practice have long been recognised, as the majority of emotional problems presented to the GP are collections of symptoms, signs and poorly defined conditions.

Jenkins et al (1985) conducted an experimental study of the classification of mental ill-health in general practice. Videotaped real life consultations concerning conditions with a psychiatric component were assessed by 27 highly experienced GPs. Written information from the patient's own GP was also available. The participants were asked to classify their diagnoses according to either the International Classification of Disease (ICD) or the International Classification of Health Problems in Primary Care (ICHPPC) criteria. The outcome was that the doctors showed extremely low diagnostic concurrence in that there was poor agreement amongst the GPs' own diagnostic labels, with a large number of unrecorded or unclassifiable responses.

In the reality of dealing with complex human behaviour, the GP is confronted with a mixed bag of symptoms for which an arbitrary disease label may or may not be helpful. For example, it is quite difficult to distinguish reliably between anxiety and depression in the general practice setting, and making the distinction may not help management decisions. But recognising the difference between clinical depression and manic-depressive illness in terms of aetiology, treatment and prognosis is essential because the management of these two conditions is very different. Acute exacerbations of manic-depressive illness may have to be referred to hospital for treatment, and clinical depression could contain elements of suicide risk. So making a diagnosis here is important.

Social causes of emotional disturbance

These factors broadly fall into four groups:

1. those concerned with acute life events
2. those that lead to chronic social stress
3. the availability and quality of social supports
4. social factors that may be thought of as risk factors.

Summary

- The majority of psychiatric problems in general practice are 'minor' psychiatric disorders.
- Most people cope with emotional disturbances given adequate social and environmental support.
- People with more severe presentations suffer for longer if undetected and untreated.
- Social and environmental factors — poverty, unemployment, social isolation, major life events, poor housing and so on — form an important part of the aetiology of mental illness.
- Social and environmental factors influence the way that people cope with major life events, including serious physical illness.

Continuing care for psychiatric problems

Primary care support for people suffering with a mental illness is available from community health services, local authority social services, general practice and voluntary agencies. The availability and accessibility of community psychiatric nurses and psychologists will determine the management of patients with both psychotic and neurotic illness. Social workers are concerned with the long-term support of those who have a chronic mental illness, and have a role in helping with some of the social factors that influence the course of mental illness.

GPs are no longer restricted to employing receptionists and nurses only. Some practices now have counsellors in their team. The effectiveness of counselling in general practice has been difficult to evaluate because of the problems in identifying satisfactory measures of outcome.

It might be helpful to think about counselling in two separate categories. The GP is familiar with giving information, explaining the meaning of diagnoses and implications of treatment, and giving advice. She or he also listens, explores the patient's feelings and difficulties, and works with them, but usually without any special training, and sometimes without the time. This latter kind of counselling could be provided by a trained counsellor, either as a crisis intervention or longer-term help.

On the whole, studies so far have found that the counsellors in general practice find their work satisfying and that GPs value their help (McLeod 1988). Community psychiatric nurses, psychologists, social workers and practice-based counsellors all have a part to play in the short- and long-term support of people who suffer mental ill-health.

Referral to specialist services

The reasons for referral to psychiatrists are complex; they include pressure from relatives and access to community services. Making a diagnosis and deciding treatment are not always the primary reasons for referral. Sometimes the GP reaches a point where management is stuck and an outside view is needed in order to progress.

Prevention of mental illness

In the main, secondary and tertiary prevention are the areas addressed in general practice psychiatry — that is, the early detection and amelioration of the consequences of the illness or treatment, the preservation or improvement of the performance of an individual's normal social role and the improvement of the quality of a person's life.

If we think about the social factors that are associated with the aetiology of mental illness, then prevention should be aimed at the reduction of risk factors such as poverty, unemployment and chronic social stress. The strengthening of protective social factors such as social support and social networks, particularly intimate or marital relationships, should reduce the impact of risk factors. Given that this is not always possible, preventive work is aimed at health education, crisis intervention, and care of vulnerable children.

Advice about alcohol consumption during health checks is an example of health education as a means of preventing alcohol-related psychological and social problems. Abortion and marital breakdown increase the risk of psychiatric illness, so counselling during these crises should help to prevent, or at least reduce, the risk of psychiatric morbidity. Marital therapy could also help to reduce the risk of emotional disturbance in children.

Practical measures in crisis intervention would be the mobilisation of social support for individuals and families, particularly following bereavement, car accidents, surgery, assaults, and similar sudden or unexpected adverse life events.

Prevention of mental ill-health in the carers of people with chronic mental illness (particularly with disabling psychotic conditions such as chronic schizophrenia, alcoholism or manic-depressive psychosis) is as important as caring for the patient. Often, spouses and children suffer the effects of living with a person with mental illness and care for them at considerable emotional cost. Their needs are not always addressed. Usually there are support groups available, for example, for the partners of alcoholics; where they are and how to find them are important pieces of information for carers.

Summary

- The major part of psychiatry in general practice is the detection, management and prevention of minor psychiatric morbidity.

- Support services from multiple agencies, including health and social services and the voluntary sector, are involved in the management of psychiatry in general practice.
- Teamwork is important for the efficient and effective delivery of services, as is good communication.

Diabetes in general practice

Until the early 1970s, diabetes was viewed very much as a chronic medical condition to be managed by the specialist. For years, medical training emphasised the specialised nature of diabetic care. GPs therefore felt neither confident nor competent to manage their diabetic patients, sending most of them to the hospital diabetic clinics. Yet, today, diabetes is a prime example of continuing care in general practice — the 'ideal disease for the general practitioner to diagnose, observe and treat with interest' (Wilkes 1973).

The details of the natural history and medical management of diabetes can be found in most medical textbooks. The information pack on diabetes produced by the Royal College of General Practitioners is particularly helpful. This section will not address the diagnosis, treatment and monitoring of diabetes, but will discuss the care of people with diabetes by general practitioners. The degree of involvement with secondary, hospital services and specialist community services will depend on the needs of the patient and how local diabetic services are organised.

The important questions in general practice diabetes include:

- Is it necessary for newly diagnosed non-insulin-dependent diabetics to attend a hospital diabetic clinic?
- Is it necessary for stable insulin-dependent diabetics to be followed up in a hospital diabetic clinic?
- Are community support services (e.g. chiropody) adequate for diabetes care?
- Is it better to monitor diabetic patients in 'mini-clinics' or normal surgery?
- What are the relative costs and benefits of mini-clinics for the patients and the practice?
- Is the GP confident and competent to manage the complications of diabetes?
- What are the continuing learning needs of GPs in relation to the management of diabetes?

Who manages diabetes?

Despite the many technical advances in the treatment of diabetes, the ultimate responsibility for managing diabetes lies with the patient, supported by their family, with a team of professional health workers performing supportive roles.

For example, when the doctor advises 'tighter glycaemic control', or the chiropodist suggests different footwear, or the dietician advises weight reduction, it is the patient who has to make adjustments in life style to achieve these outcomes. She or he has to increase the number of tablets or insulin dosage, change the times for taking the tablets or injections, buy different shoes, or change eating patterns.

The management plan

The aim of any management plan should be to enable the patient to perform their normal social role, to maintain (or improve upon) a satisfactory quality of life, and to prevent the development of secondary complications. The question of what diabetic control means needs to be examined. Shillitoe (1988) reviews a number of studies into what doctors and patients perceive to be 'control', and there appears to be a divergence of opinion. The medical profession regards the important measures of diabetic control to be the regulation of blood glucose, dietary adherence, reduction and maintenance of body weight to as close to the ideal as possible, regular taking of exercise and the control of risk factors for cardiovascular disease, such as smoking and high blood pressure. The majority of these are behavioural measures which are influenced by the patient's attitude towards self-management.

Patients, on the other hand, may be more interested in feeling good, the convenience of the management regime, avoiding sore fingers from too frequent self-monitoring of blood glucose or the social disruption of having to have meals at specific times.

The professionals are inclined to underestimate the increased social and personal demands that complicated management regimes place on the patient. For example, doctors see adherence to a dietary regime as being under the control of the patient, while patients maintain that difficulties with compliance are outside their control.

Patient education

A common assumption in poor diabetes control is that the patient does not understand the implications of poor control, or that their practical skills are inadequate. Shillitoe (1988) summarises the skills and knowledge that are needed for patients to cope with most situations.

The patient and members of the family have to become familiar with the symptoms of hypoglycaemia and hyperglycaemia. The practical skills have to be incorporated into the routines of daily living, with the family sometimes sharing special diets. Habits of a lifetime have to be changed, and all this with as little disruption to normal life as possible!

Studies of the extent of patients' knowledge of diabetes care have found serious deficiencies concerning knowledge of the natural history of diabetes and its complications, and the proficiency in practical procedures such as the use of reflectance meters and reagent strips. The reasons for this fit in with what is known about how people learn. Fears and anxieties about the disease, and general anxieties about disruption of personal, vocational and social life at the time of receiving the diagnosis make it unlikely that the patient will understand or remember unfamiliar medical concepts to do with diabetes at the time that the diagnosis is made, or during inpatient treatment.

The patient may also be overloaded with too much unfamiliar information. Shillitoe (1988) concludes that the timing of educational programmes needs to be chosen carefully, and there are 'at risk' groups of patients — such as those who are older at the time of diagnosis, the socially isolated and new referrals — who require special attention.

A number of organisations have produced guidelines for patient education programmes. The British Diabetic Association (1992) has published standards concerning clinical aspects of management and the evaluation of education as well as the content of educational programmes.

There are a wide variety of programmes aimed at individuals or groups with the objective of improving knowledge and practical skills. It must be remembered that whatever educational programme or method is selected, it will be more effective if it fits in with the patient's beliefs and attitudes about diabetes, and if the recommended regimes fit in with the cultural and traditional practices.

Necessary patient knowledge and skills

- Methods for reversing glycaemic extremes.
- Techniques for blood/urine analysis.
- Injection techniques (for IDD).
- Methods for varying and balancing diet.
- Methods for varying treatment regimes (e.g. insulin dosages).
- Accurate record keeping.

Diabetes as a tracer condition

Diabetes also qualifies as a 'tracer' for evaluating the general quality of care and the efficiency of the health care system delivering it. The idea of using 'tracer' conditions to evaluate health services was developed by Kessner in the United States (Kessner et al 1973). The tracer conditions had to be discrete, identifiable health problems, providing a framework

The tracer method — Kessner's criteria
1. A tracer should have a definite functional impact.
2. A tracer should be relatively well defined and easy to diagnose.
3. Prevalence rates should be high enough to permit the collection of adequate data from a limited population sample.
4. The natural history of the condition should vary with utilisation and effectiveness of medical care.
5. The techniques of medical management of the condition should be well defined for at least one of the following processes: prevention, diagnosis, treatment or rehabilitation.
6. The effects of non-medical factors on the tracer should be well understood.

for evaluating the interaction between patients, health care services and the environment. The tracer method also purports to measure both processes and outcomes.

Diabetes satisfies all of Kessner's criteria, and is not only a good condition for medical audit in general practice, but also for collaborative audit at the primary/secondary care interface.

The quality of diabetes care in general practice

GPs have been assuming more responsibility for their diabetic patients over the past 20 years. The trend is towards providing diabetes care in organised mini-clinics, working with other health professionals, such as practice nurses, district dieticians and/or chiropodist, opticians, and so on. Community diabetes specialists sometimes go out to GP clinics on a regular basis.

A number of GP initiatives were evaluated and published in the journals; the findings were mostly based on the outcomes of metabolic control and weight, and audits of medical records to see whether the procedures for reviewing patients were followed. It has become clear that GPs can achieve results as good as those of hospital clinics if the services are properly organised, and the team has adequate training (Hayes & Harris 1984, Singh & Holland 1984).

The GP's learning needs in diabetes

In a study of the learning needs of general practitioners in diabetes, Marsden & Grant (1990) demonstrated that most GPs were willing to spend up to 1 hour per week on updating themselves about diabetes and, furthermore, were willing to pay for it. An interesting finding, which may be common to all districts, was the GPs' perception for a need to improve clinical skills, particularly on retinal examination, adjustment of insulin or tablet therapy, and for more knowledge about dietetics.

Summary

- Diabetes is a condition which clearly illustrates the principles of continuing care in general practice.
- The responsibility for managing diabetes lies with the patient.
- Health care services for diabetes are delivered by a multidisciplinary team.
- Health education for self-management has a major role in the management of diabetes.

CONCLUSIONS

The role of the general practitioner in continuing care is multifaceted. While acknowledging that most chronic diseases cannot be 'cured', there is much to be done to alleviate suffering, and to maintain a satisfactory level of functioning. The quality of a person's life is paramount in the continuing care of any chronic condition.

Most, if not all, forms of continuing care involve more than one professional agency. The primary care team has a central role, and the value of a properly functioning team cannot be overstated. It is also important to have accurate and up-to-date information about the statutory and voluntary services that are available for supporting people with long-term disabilities living in the community.

In the final analysis, the main players in the management of chronic conditions are patients and their carers. The professionals are there in supporting roles.

REFERENCES

Baker R 1990 Care of old people; a framework for progress. RCGP Occasional Paper 45. RCGP, London
Balint M 1957 The doctor, his patient and the illness. Churchill Livingstone, Edinburgh.
Banks M H, Beresford S A A, Morrell D C, Waller J J, Watkins C J 1975 Factors influencing demand for primary medical care in women aged 20–44 years: a preliminary report. International Journal of Epidemiology 4(3): 189–195
British Diabetic Association 1992 Recommendations for diabetes health promotion clinics. BDA, London
Brooks D 1987 How to stop prescribing for acute self-limiting conditions. Update 15 August 1987: 311–317
Brumfitt W, Slater J D M 1957 Treatment of acute sore throat with penicillin. Lancet 1: 8–11
Colin-Jones D G 1988 Management of dyspepsia: report of a working party. Lancet 1: 576–578
Fitzpatrick R, Hinton J, Newman S, Scambler G, Thompson J 1984 The experience of illness. Tavistock, London
Friedman G, Siegelaub A, Seltzer C 1974 Cigarettes, alcohol, coffee and peptic ulcer. New England Journal of Medicine 290; 9: 469–473
Hayes T M, Harris J 1984 Randomised control trial of routine hospital clinics versus routine general practice care for type II diabetics. British Medical Journal 289: 728–730.
Helman C G 1984 Culture, health and illness. Wright, London
Her Majesty's Stationery Office 1983 The Mental Health Act. HMSO, London

Howie J G R 1976 Clinical judgement and antibiotic use in general practice. British Medical Journal 2: 1061–1064
Howie J G R, Hutchinson K R 1978 Antibiotics and respiratory illness in general practice; prescribing policy and workload. British Medical Journal 2: 1342
Howie J G R, Richardson I M, Gill D, Durno D 1971 Respiratory illness and antibiotic use in general practice. Journal of the Royal College of General Practitioners 21: 657–663
Jenkins R, Smarton N, Marinker M, Shepherd M 1985 A study of the classification of mental ill-health in general practice. Psychological Medicine 15:403-409
Jones R H, Lydeard S E, Hobbs F D R 1990 Dyspepsia in England and Scotland. Gut 31: 401–405
Kessner D M, Kalk C E, Singer J 1973 Assessing health quality — the case for tracers. New England Journal of Medicine 288; 4: 189–194
McCleod J 1988 The work of counsellors in general practice. RCGP Occasional Paper 37. RCGP, London
McPherson AS (ed) 1987 Women's problems in general practice. Oxford University Press, Oxford
McWhinney I R 1989 A textbook of family medicine. Oxford University Press Oxford
Marsden P, Grant V 1990 The learning needs in diabetes of general practitioners. Diabetic Medicine 7: 69–73
Meade T W, Dyar S, Browne W, Townsend J, Frank A O 1990 Low back pain of mechanical origin: randomised comparison of chiropractic and hospital outpatient treatment. British Medical Journal 300: 1431–1437
Murdoch J C 1984 Primary care for people with a mental handicap. RCGP Occasional Paper 47. RCGP, London
Roland M O, Morrell D C, Morris R W 1983 Can general practitioners predict the outcome of episodes of back pain? British Medical Journal 286: 523–525
Ross P W 1971 Accuracy of clinical assessment of microbrial aetiology of sore throat. Practitioner 207: 659
Scambler G, Hopkins A 1986 Being epileptic: coming to terms with stigma. Sociology of Health and Illness 8: 26–43
Shillitoe R W 1988 Psychology and diabetes. Chapman & Hall, London
Singh B M, Holland M R 1984 Metabolic control of diabetes in general practice clinics: comparison with a hospital clinic. British Medical Journal 289: 726–728.
Steele K, Mills, K A, Gilliland A, E W, Irwin W G Taggart A 1987 Repeat prescribing of non-steroidal anti-inflammatory drugs excluding aspirin: how careful are we? British Medical Journal 295: 962–964
Taylor R C, Buckley E G 1987 Current developments Preventive care of the elderly: a review of current developments RCGP Occasional Paper 35. RCGP, London
Tuckett D, Boulton M, Olsen C, Williams A 1985 Meetings between experts. Tavistock, London
Waddell G 1982 An approach to backache. British Journal of Hospital Medicine Sept 1982: 187–219
Whitfield M J, Hughes A O 1981 Penicillin in acute sore throat. Practitioner 225: 234–239
Wilkes J M 1973 Diabetes—a disease for general practice. Journal of the Royal College of General Practitioners 23: 46–54
Williams E I 1986 Care of old people: a framework for progress. Occasional Paper 45, British Journal of General Practice.

7. Audit and research in practice

Margaret Lloyd

Whole fields essential to the progress of medicine will remain unexplored until the general practitioner takes his place as an investigator.

Sir James Mackenzie

At the beginning of the century Sir James Mackenzie saw, and took, the opportunities for advancing our knowledge of medicine by carrying out research in his general practice in Lancashire. He invented the clinical polygraph, the forerunner of the ECG, which he used to record the pulsations of the jugular veins of his patients with the heart disease and contributed significantly to the foundation of scientific cardiology. Mackenzie's work influenced William Pickles who was to contribute so much to our understanding of the epidemiology of infectious disease (particularly infectious hepatitis) through his work in his Wensleydale practice. Since then research in general practice has developed with the establishment of the Royal College of General Practitioners' research units, university departments of general practice and the contributions of individual general practitioners. But Mackenzie's observation, with which this chapter began, is as true now as it was in 1916.

DISCUSSION POINT
Fields of research
What 'fields essential to the practice of medicine' are particularly appropriate for today's general practitioners to explore?

The aim of this chapter is to encourage you to set off on a journey of exploration and to help you to acquire some of the necessary skills for successfully completing the exploration.

RESEARCH
Why explore?

It is appropriate to liken research and audit to an exploration. Exploring a tropical forest in search of a rare animal may well be hazardous and challenging; it will certainly be expensive in terms of time and money and demands commitment. Why do some individuals do it? The reasons are likely to be complex and to vary from individual to individual. However, for the majority, an important driving force will be curiosity — the need to find out if the animal still exists and, if so, what are its habits? Finding the answer to this question is the explorer's reward and may well spur him onto further exploration. The same principles apply to audit and research.

Why undertake a research or audit project in your practice? Why not settle down to care for patients to the best of your ability without looking for further work? The problem is that you are unlikely to remain motivated and deliver the best quality care unless you develop the habit of asking questions, of 'thinking critically' as you carry out your day-to-day work. If you begin to ask questions you will want to find answers. Then you will be at the starting point of carrying out audit and research in general practice.

Starting off: selecting a question

Most explorers are motivated by their interest in a topic and by a question they feel they must answer. For Christoper Columbus this might have been 'What lies beyond the horizon?' and for Charles Darwin 'How did the numerous species of plants and animals gain their individual characteristics?'

In the same way, choosing a topic and defining the question to be answered is the starting point for all research and audit activities. Your trainer may have suggested to you that it would be a 'good thing' to do a research project in the practice. You may already have a topic which particularly interests you and a burning question you wish to answer. Probably most of you will not have reached that stage, so where do you start?

> **DISCUSSION POINT**
>
> **Starting off**
>
> Make a list of the patients you see during one or more surgeries. What problems did they present to you? Think critically about each one. What questions do they pose which you would like answered? You could make a similar list of questions following a practice meeting.

Two case vignettes

To start you off, here are two brief cases. What questions do they raise in your mind? Make a list of them.

Case 1
Mr A, aged 18 years, is a student. He was last seen in the surgery 4 years ago. He gives a 3-day history of fever, sore throat and 'feeling awful'. He complains to you that he was unable to get an appointment to see you yesterday.

Case 2
Mrs B, aged 60 years, is married to a local businessman. She is known to have non-insulin-dependent diabetes (NIDD) and receives repeat prescriptions for oral hypoglycaemics. She comes to you complaining of chest pain when she walks upstairs. She tells you that she last saw a doctor 2 years ago. 'I can't be bothered to go to the hospital — they make you wait for ages'.

Questions raised by these cases

Mr A and Mrs B present problems which are met commonly in general practice. Both of them will have raised questions for you and your list might have included the following:

Mr A
- Why is he consulting me now?
- Should I take a throat swab?
- Should I prescribe antibiotics?
- He rarely consults — is that typical of adolescents?
- Is the practice appointments system working as well as it could be?

Mrs B
- Does she have angina?
- How well is her diabetes controlled?
- She should be reviewed regularly. Why hasn't this happened?
- Why do diabetics have an increased risk of coronary heart disease?
- Are hospitals better than GPs at looking after patients with NIDD?
- Perhaps we should review the practice's repeat prescribing procedure?

Look at these questions again and think how you might group them into different categories. One way would be to group them according to the type of activity:

- *Clinical.* Should I prescribe antibiotics?
- *Epidemiological.* Why do diabetics have an increased risk of developing coronary heart disease?
- *Operational.* Could the appointments system be improved?
- *Behavioural.* Why is he consulting me now?

These four headings represent the main areas of general practice research. The second method of classification is by considering the *focus* of the question.

- The first group would include all questions focusing on the *individual patient*, e.g. does Mrs B have angina?
- The second group of questions are those which are relevant to *your practice* and the answers will be of less interest to others, e.g. is the practice appointments system working as well as it could be?
- The third group of questions are of *much wider interest*, e.g. why do patients with diabetes have an increased risk of developing coronary

heart disease? Does the taking of throat swabs improve the management of patients with sore throats?

The first group of questions form part of the everyday process of *clinical decision making*. By formulating questions or hypotheses about a patient's problems and testing them by asking further questions during the course of the consultation, we are able to make a diagnosis or produce a problem list and devise a management plan for a patient.

The second group of questions are about what is happening in your practice and what should be happening. This is the starting point of *clinical audit*.

The third group are related to our fundamental understanding of health and disease and the process of health care. They are the starting point of *research*.

Some people consider *audit* and *research* to be separate entities. In fact, they may differ in scope but they have two important features in common.

1. Audit and research projects must start with a well-defined question.
2. The method of answering the question(s) posed must be by systematic enquiry.

By now you will have realised that asking questions should be part of our everyday work. The next step is to decide on a question which you would like to answer.

What is a 'good' question?

Selecting the right question for your audit or research project is of vital importance otherwise you may waste time and effort and may eventually lose interest.

A good question is:

- *Interesting* — for you and others who may be involved. You are more likely to remain enthusiastic if the topic really 'fires' you.
- *Important and relevant* to yourself, your practice (e.g. a review of the repeat prescribing system) or to a wider audience (do diabetics have more coronary artery disease?).
- *Answerable*. Beware of being too ambitious. It is better to answer a simple question well in a relatively short period of time than get bogged down in an all-embracing question which turns out to be unanswerable.

To quote Sir Peter Medawar: 'Good scientists study the most important problem they think they can solve'.

Some would say that the question you set out to answer should be original. Certainly this applies if you are planning a research project which requires external funding. It is far less important if the project is for yourself or the practice. If it is a question *you* want to answer — go ahead.

Some handy hints

First of all develop the habit of reading journals such as the British Medical Journal and the British Journal of General Practice. This will help keep you abreast of current developments and prepare you for the MRCGP critical reading paper.

Secondly, keep a list of questions which occur to you during the course of your work. 'Sleep on them' and then weed out those which do not seem quite as good as when you first thought of them. You will probably end up with several which seem to be equally suitable for a project. You are then ready for the next step, that of looking at what others have written on the question(s) you particularly want to answer.

Exploring the literature

The next step is to read around the topic covered by your question. This will tell you:

- if your question is a reasonable one
- if others have attempted to answer it or similar questions
- about ways of approaching the question, i.e. designing an appropriate study.

There are various ways of approaching the literature.

1. The first step is to examine your question carefully and to identify some key words.

2. Then start with a few selected journals, i.e. The British Journal of General Practice, British Medical Journal and the Lancet. Take, say, the last five years and, using your key words, look through the index of relevant articles, ideally review articles which will provide you with further references.

3. To make a wider search you will need to visit a library which has the cumulative *Index Medicus* and/or the facility for computerised literature searches. Libraries which are likely to have these facilities include:

- Local postgraduate centre library — if it is of a reasonable size and employs a librarian.
- University/medical school libraries. You will be able to gain access to these via the Academic Department of General Practice (all universities and medical schools now have one).
- The Royal College of General Practitioners (see below).

Index Medicus covers the majority of the world's medical journals. Indexing is by author and subject with cross referencing. It is published each year and covers several volumes. It is wise to limit your search at first, for example to the volumes covering the last five years. The more precisely you define your key words, the easier the task will be.

The advantages of manual searches using *Index Medicus* are:

- It costs nothing.
- It allows you to discriminate between articles and select only those which are directly relevant to your question.
- It allows you to select journals which are readily accessible.

The disadvantages are:

- It is time consuming.
- You may miss relevant articles.

Computerised literature searches are now widely available in libraries. There are several data-bases, e.g. MEDLINE. The principle is the same as with manual searches using *Index Medicus*, i.e. you need carefully selected key words. Some systems will provide not only printouts of references but also abstracts of articles.

The advantages are:

- The process of searching takes less time than manual searches.
- The database may cover a wider range of journals.
- You may be able to obtain abstracts immediately — this helps you to judge the relevance of the article to your subject.

The disadvantages are:

- It costs money to use the system.
- You may be swamped by references, particularly if you have not been very selective in your choice of key words.

Services offered by the Royal College of General Practitioners

The College encourages trainees to join as associates; there is a trainee liaison officer and a trainee 'hotline' (071 823 8645). The Information Resource Centre at the RCGP provides four types of service which you may wish to use. There are charges for these services; members and associates receive discounts.

1. Enquiry service — this covers resource lists, bibliographies, practice audits and reports.
2. On-line search service, taken from either the in-house database, GP-LIT, or a commercial database, e.g. MEDLINE.
3. Library services.
4. Photocopying services, which provide photocopies of original articles.

Setting up a reference system

During your reading you will collect copies of articles and references you will wish to keep for future reference. It will make life easier if you can develop a system of keeping references which enables you to access individual articles when you need them. There are various ways of doing this — choose the one which best suits you.

If you own a computer you could set up a database of references which would allow cross referencing. Alternatively you can set up a card index of references.

Designing a study

You now have a question you wish to answer and you have read what others have written on the subject. The next step is to design a study which will enable you to answer your question:

- in a scientifically correct manner
- with the resources you have available
- in a reasonable period of time.

The planning stage is very important. Be prepared to take time over it; well thought out research is preferable to an ambitious, poorly designed study. The essential decisions to take when planning a study are:

- *Study design.* What type of study design is most suitable to answer the question?
- *Study population.* Who should be included in the study population and how should they be selected?
- *Data collection.* What data should be collected and what method of collection should be used?

What kind of study?

Studies can be either *quantitative*, involving counting and based on epidemiological methods, or *qualitative*, deriving their methodology from the social sciences.

The choice of method depends on the audit or research question you are setting out to answer. Qualitative methods are often used to explore people's attitudes or beliefs and produce small amounts of detailed information, whilst quantitative studies which often use questionnaires produce larger amounts of cruder data.

Quantitative studies. There are four types of study design (Fig. 7.1):

1. Firstly, a study which provides a snapshot of what exists *at present.* Examples:

    A. A study of the proportion of patients with diabetes who have coronary heart disease
    B. A study of patient satisfaction with the practice appointments system.

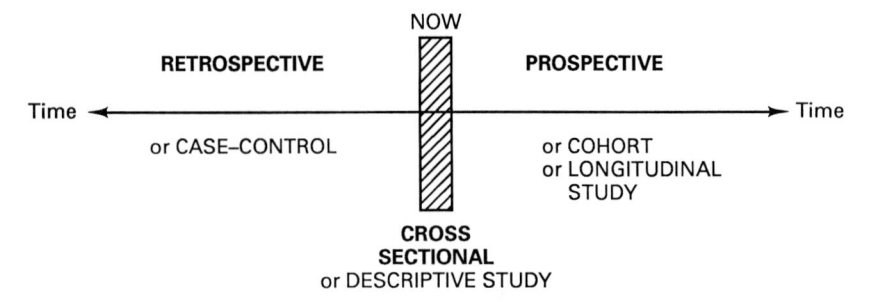

```
                        NOW
         RETROSPECTIVE    ║    PROSPECTIVE
Time  ◄──────────────────╫──────────────────►  Time
         or CASE–CONTROL  ║    or COHORT
                          ║    or LONGITUDINAL
                          ║       STUDY
                       CROSS
                     SECTIONAL
                  or DESCRIPTIVE STUDY
```

Fig. 7.1 Types of study design.

Each of these is a *cross sectional* or *descriptive* study. This is the type most commonly used in general practice audit and research.

2. Secondly, a study which looks *backwards* in time.
   Examples:

   C. The consulting patterns of adolescents over the last 5 years.
   D. A study of the relationship between smoking and coronary heart disease (CHD) in patients with diabetes.

A study to answer example C would be a retrospective descriptive study. Example D could be studied by identifying diabetics with CHD (cases) and those without evidence of CHD (controls) and comparing their smoking histories. Cases and controls should be matched in respect of their age, sex and duration of diabetes. This is an example of a *case-control* study which can provide information about factors associated with a disease relatively quickly and cheaply.

3. Thirdly, a study which looks *forward* in time.
   Example: E. a study of microalbuminuria as a risk factor for nephropathy and retinopathy in patients with diabetes.

This study would involve identifying a *cohort* of patients with diabetes, identifying those with microalbuminuria and those without, and following them over a period of time to see which ones developed diabetic complications. Several terms are used to describe this type of study, including a *longitudinal, prospective* or *cohort* study. This is a lengthier, more expensive method of determining the aetiology of a disease or its risk factors, e.g. microalbuminuria as a risk factor for diabetic complications.

4. Lastly, a study of the *effects of an intervention* of some kind. The intervention may be in the form of a drug or an activity such as providing advice about stopping smoking. Classically, as in a *clinical trial* of a new drug, one group of patients is randomly allocated to receive the drug and another group is given either a placebo or an established drug. The trial may be:

- single blind — the patient, but not the doctor, is unaware of which drug is which
- double blind — neither patient nor doctor are 'in the know'
- cross-over — the patients receive first one and then the other drug (or placebo).

Clinical trials of drugs are usually organised on a large scale by drug companies or academic institutions. General practitioners may be involved in, but rarely lead, this type of study.

Selecting the study population

Having decided which type of study is most appropriate to the question you want to answer, you will need to decide:

Whom should I study? This will obviously depend on your question. You should decide on the criteria you are going to use to both include and exclude people from the study.

Example: F. You wish to determine the morbidity of children with asthma in your practice population and have decided on the following inclusion and exclusion criteria.

— *Inclusion criteria*
- children aged 3–16 years
- a history of asthma
- children and their parents who are willing to participate.

— *Exclusion criteria*
- children aged less than 3 years
- those with other significant conditions affecting their health
- those unwilling to participate in the study.

How many people should I study? This again depends on the question you are setting out to answer, the methods you are going to use and the size of the group from which you are drawing your study population.

Examples:

G. It would be possible to study all the children with diagnosed asthma in a practice of 6000 patients (assuming 800 children aged 3–15 and an asthma prevalence of 10% — giving a study population of 80).

H. If you wished to study women's attitudes to cervical screening in a practice of 15 000 patients it would be impractical to include all women 25–65 if you were going to obtain information by inverviewing them. However, it would be possible to include them all if you were going to use a questionnaire.

Sampling It is often necessary in both research and audit to study a sample of your population. The method of sampling is very important if you are to avoid biasing your results. The first step is to identify the group from which you wish to sample. For example, you could identify all women aged 25–65 years from the practice's age-sex register or from the FHSA register. *But* remember age-sex registers are often incomplete and inaccurate.

You would then need to decide *how many* women to include in your sample. This will depend on the question you are trying to answer and the accuracy you wish to achieve. The method of calculating sample size is beyond the scope of this chapter. Details will be found in books on statistics included in the section of further reading. However, it is strongly recommended that you seek the advice of a statistician when planning a study which involves sampling.

Selecting the people to be included in your study should be done by a random method to ensure, as far as possible, that they are representative of the whole group from which the sample was taken. The best method is to use random numbers — either computer generated or from random number tables.

Other important points to remember when selecting your study population include:

1. *Defining diagnostic criteria.* This is essential if you are studying patients with a specific condition. In example F (p. 245) one of the inclusion criteria is 'History of asthma'. Who would you include? Children with a single episode of wheezing? Those with a nocturnal cough who may not have been given appropriate medication? Only those receiving treatment for asthma? It is important to specify inclusion criteria precisely.

2. *Standardising physical signs.* This is particularly important if a study is going to involve more than one GP or research worker.

Example: I. If you were planning to carry out a study of the efficacy of a new antibiotic in the treatment of otitis media, you would need to define and agree on the clinical signs, i.e. the appearance of the patient's ear drum which determines entrance to the study — pink, red, or red and bulging?

Collecting data

You may be able to use data which are already available in the practice or you may need to collect data specially for your project: it also depends on your research question.

1. Readily available data:
   - patients' notes
   - practice data, e.g. appointment books, practice nurse records, etc.
2. Specially collected data:
   - recording of practice activity on specially designed forms
   - questionnaires — these may be structured or semi-structured, self-administered or interviewer administered (see below)

- measurements, e.g. blood pressure, blood lipids, peak expiratory flow rates.

Of the specially collected information, questionnaires are probably most often used in small-scale practice audit and research studies, and their design will now be dealt with in more detail.

Designing a questionnaire Questionnaires are either self-administered (i.e. handed to the patient for them to complete) or administered by an interviewer. If you decide to use a questionnaire to collect your infomation it is essential to think carefully about the design of the questions and to try them out in a pilot study. There are several helpful books on questionnaire design available (see Further Reading).

DISCUSSION POINT

Collecting data

You have decided to find out if patients are satisfied with the practice's appointments system and to design a questionnaire to gather patients' views.

— What questions would you want to include in a questionnaire, and in what form?

Types of questions There are open and closed questions. A *closed question* forces patients to make a choice.

Example:
Would you like the surgery times to be changed?

<pre>
                    Tick one
              ☐ Yes
              ☐ No
              ☐ Don't know
</pre>

The advantage of this type of question is that the answers are easy to deal with. The disadvantage is that they provide very limited information and would not really help you to improve the system because you would not know the times preferred by the majority of patients.

The alternative is to use *open questions*.

Example:
When would you like us to hold our surgeries?

This would provide you with considerably more information than closed questions. The problem with this approach is that you are likely to get many different answers which would be difficult to deal with in the analysis.

A compromise would be to extend the closed type of question, giving patients several options.

Example:
Which would be the most convenient surgery times for you? (Tick no more than 2 boxes.)

        8.30 – 10.30 ☐
      11.00 – 12.30 ☐
        2.00 – 4.00 ☐
        6.00 – 8.00 ☐

Closed questions should be mutually exclusive otherwise confusion will arise.

Example:
How far do you live from the surgery?
    Less than 1 mile ☐
    1–2 miles ☐
    2–3 miles ☐

Which box would someone living 2 miles from the surgery tick? Better to phrase the possible responses:

    Less than 1 mile ☐
    Between 1 and 3 miles ☐
    Between 3 and 5 miles ☐

Rating scales Another method of obtaining information in a self-administered questionnaire is by using rating scales:

1. A *visual analogue scale* where the person marks a point on a line indicating their answer.

Example:
How concerned are you about your child's asthma?

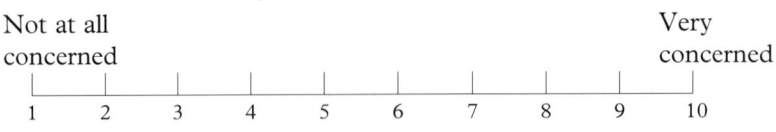

Not at all concerned   Very concerned

1 2 3 4 5 6 7 8 9 10

2. A *Likert scale* where a score is allocated to each response. This is often used to assess attitudes.

Example:
A child's asthma may be made worse by their parents smoking.

Strongly agree	Agree	Uncertain	Disagree	Strongly disagree
1	2	3	4	5

Key points to remember when designing questionnaires
- Use simple language.
- Decide whether closed or open questions, or a combination of both, are most suitable for your purposes.
- Keep the questions short and specific.

- Avoid asking leading questions.
- Avoid asking two questions in one.

Piloting your questionnaire A pilot study aims to answer the questions:

- Do patients understand the language of the questionnaire? (Comprehensibility.)
- Do they give the same answers if they complete the questionnaire on more than one occasion? (Reliability.)
- Does each question actually measure what it is designed to measure? (Validity.)

It is usually sufficient to give the questionnaire to a small number of people and then to interview them afterwards about their understanding of the questionnaire (comprehensibility) and their replies (validity).

When you have finalised your questionnaire it is time to think about how you are going to distribute it. The possible methods are:

1. By post — most postal surveys have a problem achieving more than a 60% response rate.
2. Handing it to patients when they attend the surgery.
3. Administering the questionnaire yourself or by a member of the practice team — either face to face or by telephone.

It is very important to aim for the maximum response, particularly if you are using a postal questionnaire. Ways of maximising the response include:

- a well-designed, attractively produced questionnaire
- a covering letter signed by yourself or one of the partners explaining the study and why it is important.
- enclosing an envelope for return of the questionnaire.

Using other methods of data collection It may not be appropriate to use a questionnaire to answer your audit or research question. If you are considering using one of the other methods listed there are some important points to remember.

Patients' notes and practice data Problems may arise if they are illegible and/or incomplete. Remember that you are totally dependent on what the doctor/nurse who saw the patient chose to write.

Recording of practice activity This may be done by designing a form which must be easy to fill in, particularly if it is to be completed during or after a consultation. A detailed form taking more than a minute to complete is unlikely to encourage GPs or nurses to take part in your study.

Measurements Make sure that the instruments you intend to use are reliable and accurate, and that the person using them has been adequately trained.

Always try out your method of data collection in a small pilot study.

Data handling Whichever method of data collection you use, you will inevitably end up with a lot of information which will need sorting and analysing. Data handling usually involves classifying (putting information into categories which share a common attribute) and coding (allocating a number to each category). For example, in a study of the treatment of otitis media you could use the following coding system:

Symptom	Code
Earache	1
Fever	2
Earache + fever	3

If your study has involved collecting information about patients' symptoms and diagnoses, you may wish to use a standardised classification such as the *International Classification of Primary Care* (Lamberts & Wood 1989).

Questionnaires which include closed questions are easy to code.

Example:
Which would be the most convenient surgery times for you?

		Code
8.30 – 10.30	☑	1
11.00 – 12.30	☐	2
2.00 – 4.00	☑	3
6.00 – 8.00	☐	4

Coding makes life easier if you are analysing your data by hand and is essential if you are going to use a computer. In the above example codes 1 and 3 would be punched into the appropriate computer columns.

If your questionnaire about surgery times has included a space for patients to make comments and if you wish to analyse the comments, you will need to devise your own coding system. For example, a patient may have written: 'I often find it difficult to get through to the surgery to make an appointment and would prefer it if I could just turn up on the day'. You could allocate a code to 'Preference for a non-appointment system' and another code to 'Problems with telephoning surgery' if you were wishing to look at the reasons for people's preferences in detail. If more than one person is involved in coding it is essential to check that you agree with each other by coding a small number of questionnaires and then cross checking. Always remember to record your coding system in a safe place, otherwise your computer printout or spreadsheet will mean nothing to you when you go back to it after a time.

Non-responders Whichever method of data collection you use it is very unlikely that you will be able to collect complete information from all your study population. If 65% of the patients to whom you send questionnaires actually complete it and return it to you, you have done well. But are these representative of everybody you sent them to? Perhaps elderly patients found it difficult to read and/or understand and so did not return the questionnaire. This would bias your results and could have an important effect on the conclusions you draw from your findings. It is therefore very important to look at the proportion of non-responders and to compare the information you have about them (e.g. sex, age, consultation rate, etc. obtained from practice records), with the responders to see if they are representative of the whole population.

Analysing your results This is the exciting part of research but can be daunting. If you are doing more than a small, descriptive study you will probably need help from a statistician or from one of the statistics books listed in the section on Further Reading. Focus on the questions you are aiming to answer when analysing your results.

Qualitative studies We have seen that using *closed* questions in a questionnaire limits the amount of information you can obtain. Even using *open* questions is not ideal. For example, if you wish to carry out a study looking at the reasons why some patients with diabetes default from follow-up, you could use a questionnaire which patients are asked to complete. Designing such a questionnaire would involve identifying the reasons why *you* think patients default, although you might have asked a few patients before deciding on the questions you wished to include. The problem is that you are likely to have missed out some of the possible reasons and have no way of exploring in greater depth people's reasons for non-attendance. It is in this sort of study that qualitative research methods are most useful.

The basic method of qualitative research is the interview, using semi-structured or unstructured schedules. In your study of patients with diabetes you would write down a list of topics (e.g. knowledge of diabetes, health beliefs, attitude to nurses and doctors, etc.) and then let the patient talk about each one. You would need to audiotape each interview and then transcribe it. As with quantitative studies, it is necessary to devise a method of coding the information you have obtained. This can be done by identifying the important themes which people raise during the interviews and allocating a code to each. This can be difficult as it must be done as objectively as possible.

You will appreciate that this method of research is time-consuming; the number of people you could study would need to be small and would not be representative in any way of all patients with diabetes. However, you would obtain a great deal of detailed information which would increase your understanding of why patients default. This could lead to the formation of hypotheses suitable for testing in a large-scale quantitative study.

Ethical considerations

The same ethical principles which guide clinical practice should guide research. They are:

- do good to patients (beneficence)
- do no harm (non-maleficence)
- respect patients' autonomy
- ensure confidentiality.

Translated into practical terms, the implications of the first two are clear; respecting the individual's autonomy means that *informed consent* should always be obtained from the patient, ideally in writing. Confidentiality of the information obtained must be guaranteed. If your research proposal involves studying patients it should be submitted to your local district ethical committee for approval. Your postgraduate tutor should be able to supply you with the name and address of the appropriate person to contact.

Writing a protocol

The importance of defining your research/audit question and writing down a plan of action was discussed earlier in the chapter. If you are applying for funding for your project you will need to write a formal detailed research proposal. Many grant-giving bodies provide forms and guidelines for their completion. If not, the usual headings to use in writing a proposal are:

- **Title of project**
  This should indicate what the study is about.
- **Background to the study**
  — Why did you decide to do this study?
  — What are the gaps in present knowledge?
  — How will your study contribute to knowledge and understanding in this field?
- **Aims of the study**
  — What questions are you aiming to answer?
  — What hypothesis(es) are you testing?
- **Methods**
  Study design
  Cross sectional/descriptive, case-control, longitudinal or a clinical trial?
  Study population
  — Who will be studied?
  — How are they to be selected (i.e. what are the inclusion and exclusion criteria)?
  — How many will be studied?
  — Details of sampling method if a sample is to be used.
- **Details of intervention** to be made in the case of a clinical trial, e.g. treatment.

- **Data collection**
  — What information will be collected?
  — What methods will be used?
  a) Questionnaires (self- or interviewer-administered).
  b) Interviews (semi-structured or structured).
  c) Observations to be made.
  d) Methods of measurement.
  e) Has a pilot study been carried out? If so, you should include a summary of the study, including problems encountered and changes made.
- **Data analysis**
  Give details of how data will be handled and analysed.
- **Timetable of the study**
  Set out the stages of the study and the time required for each, including the interpretation of the data and writing up the study. Be realistic and beware of setting yourself an impossible task in too short a time. It may be helpful to outline the study in the form of a flow diagram.
- **Ethical approval**
  Has it been approved by the local ethical committee?
- **References**

You may be required to produce a *summary* or *abstract* of your proposal.

Applying for funding

Research can be costly in both time and money. You may well decide that you need special funds to carry out your research project. These may be small (e.g. to cover the cost of stationery and photocopying) or large (if you need to buy protected time for yourself or an assistant).

Sources of funding

Local sources include your:

- local medical committee
- medical audit advisory group
- district health authority
- local charities
- regional health authority's locally organised research committee.

National sources of funding include:

- the Scientific Foundation Board of the Royal College of General Practitioners (apply to the RCGP for details)
- the Department of Health (DOH)
- the Medical Research Council (MRC).

It is advisable to contact the DOH or MRC for advice before applying for funding. Most organisations have deadlines for submissions of proposals and there is often a delay of several months before you receive an answer.

Another approach is to obtain a research fellowship which will enable you to spend several sessions a week carrying out your research. These are awarded by the RCGP and some departments of general practice.

Writing up your research

The fruits of your labour may be lost if you do not commit them to paper. This may be in the form of a report for yourself, for those who participated and, if appropriate, for those who funded your project. Alternatively you may decide to submit it to a medical journal — either in the form of a paper, a short report or a letter to the editor.

As a guide, structure your report or paper under the following headings:

- **Title**
- **Abstract or summary**
- **Introduction**
  Background to the study and the question you set out to answer.
- **Methods**
  How you selected your study population, collected the data and analysed the results.
- **Results**
  These are best reported in text, in tables or in diagrams. Ideally, use all three methods but make sure that you do not duplicate information in different forms.
- **Discussion**
  Aim to discuss your findings critically and in the light of what others have found. What are the main messages of your paper?
- **References**
- **Acknowledgements**

Getting your paper published

You may decide to submit your paper or short report to a journal for publication. To see your work published certainly brings satisfaction — and kudos perhaps! Some journals, e.g. the British Medical Journal, accept and publish only 20% of papers submitted. You may increase the chances of your paper being accepted by following a few simple guidelines.

- Choose an appropriate journal. Look at recent copies so that you have a good idea of the sort of papers they publish and their style.
- Read the 'Instructions to authors' which all journals publish and be careful to follow them *exactly*.
- Write a covering letter to the editor saying why you think your paper is appropriate for their journal.

If your paper is rejected by one journal, try not to be discouraged and consider submitting it to another one. The editor may ask you to revise it in the light of referees' comments and to resubmit it — very few papers are accepted without revision.

Writing a thesis for a higher degree

You may have become so enthused by your research project that you decide to write a thesis for an M Sc, M Phil or M D degree. This is not easy, particularly if you are in full-time general practice. But don't be discouraged! Read the regulations for higher degrees of your university and discuss it with a member of your local academic department of general practice. It may be possible to apply for study leave at some stage during your research.

Checklist for a trainee research project

- Define your area of interest.
- Formulate the research question.
- Carry out a literature search.
- Background reading.
- Discuss the project with your trainer and other appropriate advisers (e.g. a statistician if your project is more than a simple descriptive study).
- Reformulate the research question if necessary.
- Decide what type of study will answer your question.
- Decide who you are going to include in your study (study population).
- What data will be collected?
- How are you going to collect it?
- Carry out a pilot study to test methods.
- How will the data be handled and analysed?

    INTO ACTION!

- Analyse your results.
- Write up your project.
-     WELL DONE!

AUDIT

This section of the chapter will concentrate on audit; we shall look at the reasons for doing audit, how to select a topic and how to carry out a practice-based audit.

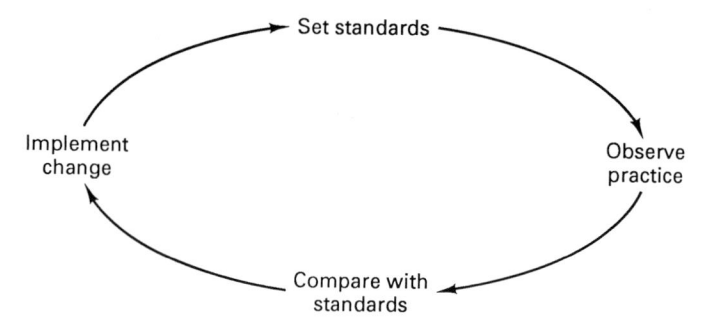

Fig. 7.2 The audit cycle.

What is audit?

Audit is concerned with quality of care. In some ways it is an unfortunate choice of name because of its association with accountancy and monitoring. 'Quality assurance' is better and is widely used in North America. Other terms which are used and have a similar meaning to audit include 'performance review' and 'peer review'.

Medical audit can be defined as:

The systematic critical analysis of the quality of medical care.

The essential features of audit have been summarised as a cycle (Fig. 7.2). However, this does not illustrate the continuous nature of audit. The 'audit spiral' (Fig. 7.3) has been suggested as a more appropriate term.

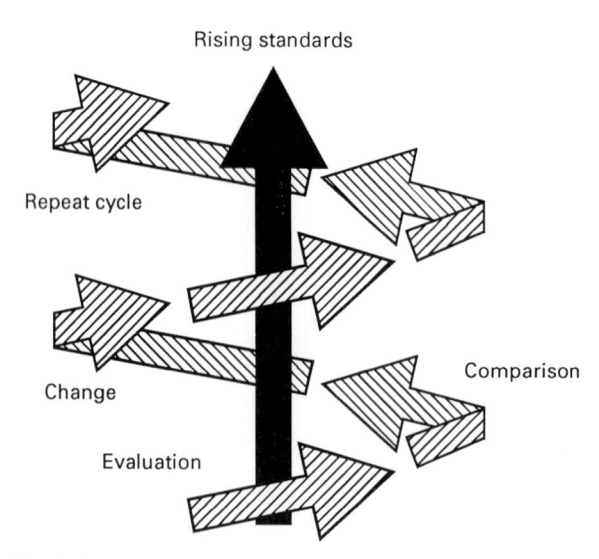

Fig. 7.3 The audit spiral.

Audit shares many of the features of research. The essential differences are:

1. Audit involves the setting of standards and comparing these with observed practices.
2. The results of audit are usually of local rather than widespread interest.

A brief history of audit

The critical evaluation of health care began in the USA in the 1950s. In this country the issues of standard setting and performance review in general practice were addressed by the Royal College of General Practitioners in their Quality Initiatives in the 1980s (RCGP 1985). The aim was to raise the quality of care in general practice. This initiative stimulated many practices to carry out audit but these were in the minority. The NHS reforms of 1990 aimed to get every practice auditing and set up medical audit advisory groups (MAAGs) in every FHSA to facilitate audit. Concern was expressed within the profession that this was a move towards imposed external audit, e.g. the monitoring of doctors' performance by an external body. This concern has not been realised and emphasis has been placed on audit being an educational process and being profession-led. This has been central to the work of the MAAGs, who ensure confidentiality of the information they gather.

Why carry out audit?

Our medical training does not help us to embrace audit with enthusiasm. We are not encouraged to identify and analyse the errors we make, and we

---

Reasons for carrying out audit

Overall:
- To improve the quality of patient care.

More specifically:
- To identify areas where improvement is necessary in:
— clinical care
— practice organisation.
- To facilitate the changes necessary for improvement.
- To educate, stimulate and enthuse the practice team.
- To increase resources
— financial
— people
— local services.

too often learn to associate error with blame. This negative approach is compounded by viewing audit as a monitoring rather than an educational process. In adopting a more positive attitude to audit it may help to look at the positve reasons for doing audit and to concentrate on the benefits it can bring.

> **DISCUSSION POINT**
>
> *Reasons for audit*
>
> Your trainer has suggested that you carry out an audit project in the practice during your trainee year. Think about how you would decide:
>
> — What to audit.
>
> — How to carry out the audit.
>
> — How you would use the results of the audit in the practice.

How to carry out an audit

First of all, audit does not have to be complicated, and the aim for your first audit should be to *keep it short and simple* (KISS). It is essential to have a well-defined question arising from an identified problem in the practice and a well-thought-out plan of action. This should be written down and discussed within the practice. It is important that all members of the practice team who are likely to be affected by the audit know about it and have the opportunity to contribute to the plan. The results and their implication for the practice must be shared with all members of the team. Some guidelines for planning an audit are shown on page 259.

Choosing a topic for audit

The most important point to remember is that the topic you choose should represent *a problem* which is important to the practice team and which they wish to solve. Additional points to consider are:

- Is it likely to benefit patients?
- Is it likely to benefit the practice?
- Is it important in professional development?
- Is it likely to repay the effort, time and money invested in the project?
- Is it of sufficient interest and importance to the practice team to maintain their enthusiasm?

The topic you choose is likely to be in one of four categories:

- clinical care
- prescribing

PRACTICE AUDIT — HOW TO DO IT

1. **Background**
   As a starting point it is helpful to clarify the problem which initiated the audit.
2. **Define the questions you wish to answer**
   i.e. What are the aims of the audit?
3. **Set criteria and standards**
   'Ideally, what should be happening?'
4. **Decide on the method to be used for observing what is happening**
   — How will the information be collected?
   — From whom?
   — By whom?
5. **Collect the information**
6. **Analyse the results**
7. **Compare results** with the standards set
8. **What needs to be changed?**
9. **How can we implement change?**

- preventive activities
- practice organisation.

When choosing a topic it is helpful to think of the care we provide for patients under the three headings of *structure, process* and *outcome*, each of which can be audited. As an example, an audit of the care of patients with diabetes could look at the following aspects of care:

Auditing the structure, process and outcome of diabetic care

STRUCTURE

Definition: The facilities available for providing care e.g. the building, people, equipment, etc.

Example: Availability of:
— urine- and blood-testing equipment
— facilities for fundoscopy
— a register of diabetic patients.

PROCESS

Definition: The use which is made of the facilities, i.e. what is actually done.

Example: The proportion of diabetic patients who have had their fundi/feet/blood pressure examined during the past year.

OUTCOME

Definition: The changes in patients' health status which can be attributed to care given.

Examples:
- Level of diabetic control.
- Number of patients in practice admitted to hospital with diabetic ketosis or hypoglycaemia during a fixed period of time.

- Number of patients developing diabetic complications over a fixed period of time.
- Level of patient satisfaction with the service provided.

> **DISCUSSION POINT**
>
> **Topics for audit**
>
> Look back at the two case vignettes of Mr A and Mrs B (p. 238). Imagine that you have seen them in your practice. Think again of the questions they raised for you.
>
> — Which ones might be suitable for an audit project?

Methods of audit

Two of the essential features of audit are:

- observation of what is happening in the practice
- comparison of these observations with a standard, i.e. what should be happening.

Observing current practice

This usually, but not always, involves collecting numerical information. Sources of data for audit include:

- routine practice data
- medical records
- practice activity analysis
- surveys — using questionnaires
- recording of specific data prospectively.

It is important to remember that audit does not necessarily involve counting. A good example is the confidential enquiry into perioperative deaths (CEPOD) which is based on case analysis. In general practice, the detailed, critical study of individual cases can provide valuable information on the quality of care provided and identify areas where change is necessary. Cases may be selected randomly or may be defined by a common characteristic (e.g. patients presenting with abdominal pain or patients referred to a dermatologist in the last six months). Case analysis can also be used when unexpected, undesirable events occur in the practice.

Mr S, aged 40 years, dies suddenly in the night during an acute attack of asthma. Everyone in the practice is understandably concerned as they consider that Mr S's death may have been avoidable. They decide to carry out a detailed study of Mr S's notes and the circumstances surrounding his death. Their findings include the following:

- Mr S had last attended the surgery 2 years previously. He had been receiving repeat prescriptions for Ventolin inhalers.

Previously he had been under the care of the local hospital and it was assumed that he was attending the asthma clinic there; in fact he had defaulted. As a result of this case study the practice decided to draw up an asthma protocol, to set up a register of patients with asthma, to change their repeat prescribing system and to look at the feasibility of setting up an asthma clinic.

This form of audit, which is qualitative rather than quantitative, can be carried out by individuals, by the doctors in a practice, or by all members of the primary health care team and can lead to a significant improvement in the quality of care.

Setting criteria and standards

This is often a difficult part of audit. First of all, what do we mean by a criterion and a standard? As an example, consider the care of patients with diabetes. This can be thought of as a series of building blocks which would include making the correct diagnosis, regular reviewing of clinical parameters and providing the patient with support and education. Which of these could be used to assess the quality of care? You could say 'all of them', but a criterion must be *measurable* and it would be difficult to measure the support you give patients. Two possible ways would be to say that there should be:

- regular monitoring of patients' blood glucose and glycolysated haemoglobin levels
- regular examination of their fundi.

But these statements are not precise enough; what is meant by 'regular' — every 6 weeks, 6 months or two years? We could say that *annual* fundoscopy is an indicator of the quality of care of patients with diabetes. This is a *criterion* of diabetic care. A *criterion* is a measurable aspect of care or practice that can be used to assess quality. A *standard* describes the level of care to be attained in the practice for any particular criterion. For the example of diabetic care this might be that 70% of patients with diabetes in the practice should have annual fundoscopy. In an audit spiral, once a standard is achieved it should then be set at a higher level.

How are criteria selected and standards set? There are two sources.

- *External standards*, which are set by a body outside the practice, e.g. the cervical screening and immunisation targets.
- *Internal standards* — these are set by the practice, usually after someone has studied the relevant literature and maybe asked the experts and colleagues.

There is evidence to suggest that standards, as with guidelines and protocols, are more likely to be achieved and adhered to if they are drawn up and 'owned' by members of the practice.

Implementing change

The focus of audit must be on improving the quality of patient care. Collecting data and setting standards will not in themselves improve quality. This will only happen if the gap between 'What we are doing' and 'What we should be doing' is progressively narrowed. This involves identifying the reasons for the gap and looking at ways in which it can be closed.

In the majority of practices patient care involves a team of people; it is unlikely that changes will be made successfully unless each member of the team is 'on board' the train of change. Remember that patients also may need to be on board. Making changes may require greater skill than achieving the other steps of the audit spiral. It is difficult to complete one turn of the spiral, but patient care will not necessarily improve unless this happens.

Does audit work?

Large amounts of money are being spent on audit. Is this money well spent? Will it lead to an improvement in the quality of care of patients? Instinctively one feels that it should do, but very little research has been done in this area. The North of England Study of Standards and Performance in General Practice (1992) was a large, ambitious study which set out to answer this question. Standards for the management of a number of common childhood conditions were set by participating groups of general practitioners, and their subsequent management of patients measured against these standards. The results of the study showed a shift in management towards the standards set, with the greatest change being observed in the doctors who had been involved in standard setting. This suggests that the process of audit, and standard setting in particular, can produce desirable change. However, it must be remembered that the doctors involved in the study were all trainers and hence not representative of all general practitioners. The honest answer to 'Does audit work?' must be 'We don't know', but this must not deter us from critically evaluating what we do in practice.

SUMMARY

1. Research answers the question 'What is right?'. Audit answers the question 'Is what I am doing right?'.
2. Successful research and audit starts with a good, well-defined question.
3. A good question is:

- interesting
- important and relevant
- answerable within a reasonable period of time.

4. The main areas of general practice audit and research are:
    - clinical
    - epidemiological
    - operational
    - behavioural.

5. Audit aims to improve the quality of patient care by comparing what is being done against a standard and correcting identified deficiencies. Audit does not have to be complicated in order to improve care.

REFERENCES

Lamberts H, Wood M 1989 ICPC International Classification of Primary Care. Oxford University Press, Oxford
North of England Study of Standards and Performance in General Practice 1992 Medical audit in general practice I: effects on doctors' clinical behaviour for common childhood conditions. British Medical Journal 304: 1480–1484
RCGP 1985 What sort of doctor? Assessing quality of care in general practice. Report from General Practice 23. RCGP, London

FURTHER READING

QUESTIONNAIRE DESIGN

Bennett A E, Ritchie K 1975 Questionnaires in medicine: a guide to their design and use. Nuffield Provincial Hospital Trust, Oxford University Press, Oxford (A short comprehensive manual)
Sudman S, Bradburn N 1983 Asking questions. Jossey Bass (Comprehensive textbook covering most of the problems and pitfalls that are likely)

EPIDEMIOLOGY AND STATISTICS

Bland M 1987 An introduction to medical statistics. Oxford University Press, Oxford
Campbell M J, Machin D 1990 Medical statistics. A common sense approach. J Wiley & Son, Chichester
Morrell D 1988 Epidemiology in general practice. Oxford University Press, Oxford (Good introduction to epidemiology based on examples drawn from general practice).
Sackett D L, Haynes R B, Guyatt G H, Tugwell P 1991 Clinical epidemiology; a basic science for clinical medicine. Little, Brown & Co, Boston (A classic text; not an easy read but well worth the challenge).

ETHICS

British Medical Association 1988 Philosophy and practice of medical ethics. British Medical Association, London

AUDIT

Baker R 1988 Practice assessment and quality of care. Occasional paper no 39. The Royal College of General Practitioners, London
Baker R, Presley P 1990 The practice audit plan — a handbook of medical audit for primary care teams. Severn Faculty of the Royal College of General Practitioners, Canynge Hall, Bristol BS8 2PR (Brief and inexpensive. A 'how to do it' guide).

Hughes J, Humphrey C 1990 Medical audit in general practice: a practical guide to the literature. Kings Fund Centre for Health Services Development, London (An excellent review of the literature).

Irvine D H 1990 Managing for quality in general practice. King Edward's Hospital Fund for London (An introduction to quality assurance in practice).

Irvine D, Irvine S (eds) 1991 Making sense of audit. Radcliffe Medical Press, Oxford (A very good, practical introduction to audit).

Marinker M (ed) 1990 Medical audit and general practice. British Medical Journal & MSD Foundation, London (A substantial, thought-provoking introduction to audit).

Sheldon M G 1988 Medical audit in general practice. Butterworth prize essay 1982, Occasional paper no 20. The Royal College of General Practitioners, London (An excellent introduction to the principles and practice of audit).

RESEARCH METHODS

Armstrong D, Calnan M, Grace G 1989 Research methods for general practice. Oxford University Press, Oxford

Howie J G R 1989 Research in general practice, 2nd edn. Chapman & Hall, London (Both of these books provide a good introduction to research methods in general practice).

Moser B A, Kalton G 1986 Survey methods in social investigation. Gower, London (A good reference text).

WRITING A PAPER

O'Connor M 1991 Writing successfully in science. Chapman & Hall, London

SECTION 3

The MRCGP and other examinations

8. The MRCGP examination

Joe Rosenthal

INTRODUCTION

One thing all of us who have been through medical training have in common is a love/hate relationship with examinations. As a GP trainee, you are in a position to acquire a whole string of letters after your name by sitting exams for the various diplomas and certificates on offer. Indeed, a condition probably unique to trainees has been lightheartedly described and given the nama 'diplomatosis'. Although this condition is rarely fatal and usually self-limiting, it can have serious complications in terms of your time, your social life, and your bank balance; more to the point, it may have a major influence on the breadth of the educational experience you get from your general practice training.

There are some clear benefits to taking exams. They stimulate reading and increase knowledge in the subject area, and (if passed) may increase self-esteem and boost career prospects. But, as has already been suggested, there is a cost in terms of money, time and emotional strain. The message is simply to consider which exams you wish to embark upon within the broader context of your overall training and personal development.

In this chapter we shall focus on the examination for membership of the Royal College of General Practitioners (MRCGP); Chapter 9 outlines some of the other popular exams for trainees.

Background to the examination

The MRCGP is now a well-established and respected examination. Every year about 2000 candidates enter. Its aim is 'to provide a framework for preparation for practice and encourage systematic reading, study and discussion'. If you are only going to go for one postgraduate qualification then this is the one to aim for. It has been suggested that passing this exam may in the future become a requirement for entry into general practice, but this is not at present the policy of the Royal College of General Practitioners or any other body. Why then do so many doctors enter? A questionnaire survey of 280 trainees has shown that 71% saw the examination as a help in getting a job, 67% as a personal hurdle or discipline, and 66% considered that its most important role was to ensure a basic level of competence before supervision ceased (Tombleson & Wakeford 1989).

The Royal College has gone to great lengths to monitor continuously the reliability and validity of its exam and publishes much information to enable interested outsiders to judge its adequacy. Examiners are carefully selected by a standard process which includes them taking the written papers and achieving a satisfactory mark. Their performance is also continuously assessed, both by direct observation and by videotape recording. Each year, in addition to examining twice, examiners attend a three-day workshop where questions are refined and new developments in the examination are discussed. For a thorough review of the background to the exam and helpful analysis of the papers it is worth obtaining Occasional Paper 46 (Lockie 1990) from the RCGP.

The examination takes place twice a year, with candidates sitting the three written papers in one of 12 centres (10 in the UK as well as one in Eire and one in Germany). Candidates who achieve marks above a certain level (one standard deviation below the mean) are invited to attend an oral examination six weeks later in either London or Edinburgh. The three written papers and two orals each contribute 20% of the total marks.

The syllabus

The content of the examination is based upon the content of general practice as defined in *The Future General Practitioner — Learning and Teaching* (RCGP 1972). See Appendix I for the detailed syllabus. Note that it is described in terms of different areas of knowledge, skills and attitudes.

Eligibility

The regulations state that candidates must be fully registered medical practitioners who have completed, or who will complete within eight weeks of the date of the oral examination, three years' full-time, or equivalent part-time, post-registration experience which includes:

(i) not less than two years in general practice (including any periods as a trainee practitioner), or
(ii) one year as a trainee practitioner and two years of full-time medical experience all within the United Kingdom and Eire, or as specially recognised by the College.

Application

The examination takes place each May and October with the orals following about six weeks later. Application forms are obtained from The Examination Department, The Royal College of General Practitioners, 14 Princes Gate, London SW17 1PU (telephone 071-581 3232), and must be submitted not less than seven weeks before the date set for the written part of the examination. The details of how to apply are published at intervals in the *British Journal of General Practice*, or an explanatory booklet may be obtained from the RCGP. The application fee at the time of writing is £290. Try to regard this as an investment in your future and it won't seem so bad. In fact, this amount barely covers the examination department's expenses in running the complex process smoothly and efficiently.

With the application form, you will be sent a set of instructions including:

- The dates and venues for the written part of the examination.
- A booklet describing the various parts of the examination.
- The procedures and papers required for obtaining the certificates in cardiopulmonary resuscitation (CPR) and child health surveillance (CHS). A candidate must have these certificates before taking the rest of the examination.
- A set of sample past question papers from the membership examination.

The introduction of the requirement for evidence of competence in cardiopulmonary resuscitation was a response to evidence that junior hospital doctors were not proficient in these techniques (Lowenstein et al 1981, Skinner et al 1985), which have been shown to save lives in some emergency situations likely to involve GPs (Vincent et al 1984, Pai et al 1987). The certificate is obtained by attending a training session by one of the authorities approved by the College. Addresses are provided when you apply for the exam. The certificate in child health surveillance is a new requirement at the time of writing and is intended to make the MRCGP a qualification for FHSA approval to carry out CHS. Certification for CHS is obtained by undertaking satisfactorily each of the listed, required procedures under supervision of either:

a. a principal in general practice undertaking child health surveillance on a regular basis and approved to do so by the relevant FHSA or appropriate body, or
b. other doctors currently undertaking child health surveillance under the auspices of a local district health authority or appropriate body.

So, in order to apply for the exam, you will need to send in the following:

- completed application form, endorsed, if you are within one year of completing vocational training, by your postgraduate dean, regional advisor, associate advisor in general practice or course organiser
- examination fee
- photocopy of your current GMC certificate of registration
- certificates attesting competence in CPR and CHS.

The examination format

The examination is in two parts. The first consists of three written papers which are completed on the same day:

a. a multiple choice question paper (MCQ)
b. a modified essay question paper (MEQ)
c. a critical reading question paper (CRQ).

The critical reading paper was introduced in 1990, replacing the traditional essay question (TEQ), also sometimes referred to as the practice topic question (PTQ) with its three compulsory essays, which you will find in earlier past papers.

The second part consists of two consecutive oral examinations held approximately six weeks after the written papers. Invitation to the oral examination is dependent on reaching a sufficient total mark in the written papers. Oral 1 is based on the candidate's Practice Experience Questionnaire (log diary) and Oral 2 on a general mixture of clinical problems and topics from general practice, often based on situations which the examiners have personally experienced.

The results are published in the week following the last oral examination when a list is posted at the College and each candidate informed of their result by post. Results will not be given over the telephone. The result may be pass, pass with distinction (for an overall mark of greater than 70%), or fail. You will receive a breakdown of your marks for each paper, and a medal is awarded to the candidate who achieves the highest overall mark of the year. The usual pass rate is in the region of 70%.

The multiple choice question paper (MCQ)

The time allowed for this paper is two hours. It is designed to test factual knowledge about all areas in which an ordinary well-informed general practitioner could be expected to have a working knowledge.

Until recently, there have been 60 questions, each question consisting of a statement, or stem, followed by five completions or items. Each item could be answered 'true' or 'false' or 'don't know'. One mark was awarded for a correct answer, none for a 'don't know' and minus one mark for an incorrect answer. From October 1992 the format has changed. The new paper still comprises questions of the true/false type but the number of items per question will vary between three and six. The total number of items will be 360 and the number of question stems may therefore vary. With the aim of rewarding achievement rather than penalising ignorance, the negative marking system has been abolished and candidates are now awarded one mark for each item correctly identified as true or false. Marks are no longer deducted for incorrect answers or for failure to answer. The total score on the paper will be the number of correct answers given, and so it is advisable

Table 8.1 Balance of questions in the MCQ

Subject area	Items
Medicine	60
Therapeutics	36
Surgical diagnosis	18
Physical medicine/trauma	18
Infectious diseases	12
Care of the elderly	12
Paediatrics	30
Psychiatry	36
Obstetrics/Gynaecology	36
Dermatology	24
Ophthalmology	18
ENT	12
Ethical/legal	12
Epidemiology/research methods	12
Practice organisation	24

to attempt all items. The paper now also contains a small number of untested items included for trial purposes but these are disregarded in the calculation of a candidate's score.

The balance of questions is subject to change but, at present, the number of items in each subject area is approximately as shown in Table 8.1.

Questions are not grouped by subject on the examination paper and may appear in any order.

Preparation and approach

The MCQ is the written paper which tends to cause the most pessimism amongst candidates. It seems an impossible task to prepare for such a global test of knowledge, but do not despair! The exam is not designed to catch you out on obscure points but to test your general grasp of basic issues arising in practice. Although original past papers are not provided, since the College must protect its pool of questions, many practice papers are available and these are well worth working through, not only to improve your techniques but also to identify and make up for gaps in your knowledge. Try to approach each paper as an exam and resist the temptation to refer to answers before you reach the end.

On the day, candidates almost always find the paper less difficult than those they have practised with. This is probably because you can never really reproduce the motivation and adrenaline needed to search your knowledge base thoroughly in the artificial situation.

Be sure to read the questions carefully. This is standard advice but cannot be repeated too often. Exact wording makes all the difference. There are some conventional terms which the examiners define in the notes on the examination which you will receive with your application form:

- *'Characteristic'* implies a feature of diagnostic significance whose absence would cast doubt on the diagnosis.
- *'Typical'* implies a feature whose presence would be expected but is perhaps not so diagnostically absolute as 'characteristic'.
- *'Recognised'* implies a fact which has been reliably reported and which a candidate would be expected to know, without the fact being necessarily characteristic or typical.
- *'Has been shown'* implies information which has been repeated so often as to gain the accolade of accepted truth or could be demonstrated by reference to an authoritative paper on the subject.
- Beware *'always'*, *'never'* and *'usually'*.

You have probably already developed an approach to MCQs which suits you. There is no one right way to do it. It is probably a good idea, however, to go through the paper initially answering those questions which you can deal with confidently, and then return to the ones which require more thought. The new marking system has ended the debate as to whether it is worth making an educated guess. Every question should now be attempted.

The modified essay question paper (MEQ)

The time allowed for this paper is now two hours (previously 90 minutes). It is designed to test problem solving, decision making and management. It looks not just at what knowledge you have got, but how you use it in situations which might arise at any time in practice.

The MEQ type paper was first developed for the MRCGP and has since been widely adopted in undergraduate and postgraduate medical education, both as a formal assessment method and as an aid to learning. It has been thoroughly researched and refined by the College over the years since its introduction.

The 'traditional' MEQ has consisted of a set of eight to ten questions which gradually unfold a story relating to a central patient and/or family — thus, it was thought, simulating the time scale and complexity of general practice. This is the sort of question you will find in the past papers prior to 1987. It has since been appreciated by the examiners that now that the majority of candidates are trainees, these sort of scenarios are not representative of their everyday experience, and so recent papers have tended to present a set of discrete problems, such as might arise in a typical surgery or a day in practice.

The paper is presented as a set, usually of ten situations, each printed on a separate page. The space below and over the page is left for your answer to a short question, usually of an open type such as 'What issues does this presentation raise?' or 'Outline your management'.

Occasional Paper 46 (Lockie 1990) describes a number of recurrent themes from the last ten years' MEQ papers. These include:

- clinical medicine, including chronic illness, prescribing, and preventive medicine
- 'problem' patients, whose personalities, expectations, circumstances and life styles may affect management
- psychological problems of individuals and families, and their treatment
- the consultation process and dynamics
- general practice organisation, including the primary health care team and problems of practice administration
- relationships with other medical and paramedical colleagues
- controversial and 'hot' topics, e.g. alcohol, AIDS, alternative medicine, environmental medicine
- the doctor's own feelings, stresses and self-awareness
- ethical and attitudinal issues.

Each question is marked by one examiner, with a 5–10% random sample of scripts re-marked by a senior examiner to check consistency. The marking schedule is prepared at the annual examiners' workshop and a fairly rigid marking grid is produced for each question. It will be useful if you bear in mind that the usual marking schedule divides the marks for each question into five groups of nine points. Each group deals with one or more aspects of the question. Thus, to gain a high score you need to deal with at least five issues per question. There are some discretionary marks available for especially comprehensive answers.

Preparation and approach

The MEQ aims to reflect practice, and so the best preparation is to see a lot of patients, think carefully about your management and discuss problems with your trainer and members of your half-day release course. It is also immensely valuable to work through old MEQs, both alone and with colleagues. You will receive some papers from the College but there are also several books of examples, often with model answers given. Always read the questions carefully and think in broad terms from all the different viewpoints, i.e. doctor, patient, family, practice team, community and so on. Be wary of suggesting just one course of action, always consider *options*, with the advantages and disadvantages of each one.

There are a number of aides-memoire which you can bear in mind for answering questions, but examiners are aware of these formulae and you should avoid appearing like a 'course clone' and sticking rigidly to structures which may not apply to all questions. The following suggestions may help you to devise your own checklists to use when answering MEQs. When asked a question on management of a situation, consider the problem in terms of its physical, psychological and social aspects. Remember, management does not just mean treatment but includes clarifying the problem by exploring the individual's past history, their ideas, concerns and expectations and any physical examination or investigation which may be indicated. The options for action once the problem is clarified might include advising and counselling, prescribing, referring, performing a procedure, or observing for a time. Try to include in your mental checklist prevention, education, ethical issues and confidentiality. When considering referral, remember that this may be within the primary health care team, to hospital services, social services or self-help and voluntary agencies. Before you leave a problem, check that you have considered liaison and follow-up and checked the patient's understanding of the situation.

Divide your time evenly between the questions, this will usually mean 12 minutes each. It is worth spending a couple of minutes planning your answer before you put pen to paper. Write clearly and in note form with liberal use of headings and underlining. It is much easier to pick up marks in this way rather than using continuous prose. Don't be afraid of repeating yourself in different questions since they will be marked separately.

With a logical approach and some lateral thinking, you can pick up a lot of marks in the MEQ. If you enjoy general practice, you can enjoy preparing for, and even sitting, this part of the exam.

The critical reading question paper (CRQ)

The time allowed for this paper is two hours, plus an additional 15 minutes to read the written material presented. It is designed to test the candidate's skills in understanding, summarising and critically evaluating written material encountered in general practice and their ability to apply what has been read.

The main way general practitioners keep up-to-date is still through reading, and with the ever-growing volume of written material available it is essential to develop skills in dealing with this literature selectively and critically. The College examiners have long felt anxiety that many candidates were unable to relate their clinical decisions to major published works (Belton 1986), and this paper has been developed in response to their concern. Appraisal skills are tested not just for dealing with articles published in 'learned' journals but also written material you might come across in everyday work, such as letters from colleagues and patients, drug advertisements, practice protocols and audits.

The paper normally contains three questions, all of which must be answered. Marks are divided equally between the questions.

Question 1 is usually in three parts and sets out to test critical appraisal skills. You are presented with a published paper from an established medical journal (minus its abstract). You will be asked to list the main points made in the article, comment on aspects of the design of the study and then discuss the implications and application of the results to general practice.

Question 2 is in three parts and tests familiarity with published literature in areas of current interest in general practice. Examples of issues addressed in previous papers include the treatment of mild hypertension, GP diabetic care, surveys of GPs' preparedness to deal with HIV and AIDS, surveillance of the elderly, management of acute MI in general practice, and mammographic screening for breast cancer.

Question 3 is in two parts and again tests critical appraisal. You are presented with, and asked to analyse and respond to, a piece of written material such as might be commonly encountered in practice. Previous examples include a letter from a Public Health Consultant regarding a local upsurge in cases of meningococcal meningitis, and a draft practice protocol for management of acute asthma.

As you will have gathered, the CRQ has a total of eight parts. Each part has a maximum of seven marks and a minimum of one. Marks are awarded for demonstrating factual knowledge and mentioning references but the majority of points will be gained by showing that you have read and understood relevent literature on the subject.

Preparation and approach

Once again, practise past questions when you can.

For the first part of this paper you need to develop your skills in appraising articles in the journals. A number of books can help you with this (see Ch. 10); probably the most comprehensive guide is the chapter 'How to read a clinical journal' in Sackett's book *Clinical Epidemiology* (Sackett et al 1991). We have prepared a 'crib' to provide a framework to try when you read a scientific article (see Appendix II). You might like to use this as a basis to develop your own checklist which you can then start to apply to any papers you read. We would highly recommend that you get together with a group of colleagues who are also preparing for the exam and present to each other some papers you have read, criticising them in this way. This serves the dual purpose of practice in appraisal and learning from other people's reading.

The first part of question 1 often amounts to a request to write an abstract for the paper you have been given. To do this, have in mind a set of headings such as those used, for example, in the 'Papers' section of the British Medical Journal, i.e.:
- objectives
- design
- setting
- subjects
- interventions (if relevant)
- main outcome measures
- results
- conclusions.

Candidates are often anxious about how much epidemiological method and statistics they need to know for this paper. A detailed grasp of statistics is an elusive thing, and for many of us only seems to come when you have a need to use it yourself as a tool for preparing your own studies. It is not difficult, however, to gain a basic understanding of the principles such as probability and validity which you need to criticise a paper. Make sure you get to grips in particular with principles of different study designs, subject selection, significance level, p values, the t-test and the chi-square test.

In preparing for question 2 of the CRQ, there is really no substitute for reading the literature. We will discuss later how you might realistically approach this task. You will gain marks for any references you can give in detail (main author and year where possible), but in order to pass you do not need to be the human equivalent of *Index Medicus*! The bulk of the marks are gained for showing that you have read and understood the important literature on the subject. Above all else, do not omit relevant information merely because you can't quote its source; there is no negative marking in this paper. Again, meeting occasionally with colleagues and discussing papers you have read is invaluable and enjoyable preparation.

Question 3 of the CRQ is not one that has any specific material to prepare with. Each day in practice you will have been dealing with the various forms of written material in your in-tray and considering your options for dealing with it. A useful exercise from time to time is to sit down with your trainer or another colleague and work your way together through their incoming mail.

On the day, plan your time for each part of the question. Allow 15 minutes for each of the eight parts and plan your answers before you write.

The oral examination

Candidates are invited to the oral examination on the basis of performance in the written papers. Only those scoring more than one standard deviation below the mean are excluded. This means that over 80% go through. Oral examinations take place at the College itself in London and at the Royal College of Physicians in Edinburgh. You will specify your preferred venue when you apply for the exam. There are two half-hour vivas with an interval of approximately ten minutes. Each viva attracts 20% of the overall marks for the membership. In each one, there are two examiners who question you alternately. There will sometimes be an observer or video camera to monitor the performance of the examiners. Before the oral, you will have completed and sent in a Practice Experience Questionnaire (log diary) with details of your practice and a log of 50 patient contacts. This provides the basis of the first viva. The second viva is based on planned questions and covers the whole range of general practice. The examiners are not aware of your marks in the written papers but do take into account subjects already covered in the previous parts of the exam.

The examination board of the College has gone to great lengths over the years to refine the oral part of the MRCGP and make it as valid and reliable as possible. They have emphasised that the aim of the oral is not to assess factual knowledge but rather to judge the candidate's approach to practice and the justification of that approach. They have identified seven areas of competence which have been used to make a marking grid for each viva. These areas are as follows:

- problem definition
- management
- prevention
- practice organisation
- communication
- professional values
- personal and professional growth.

Examiners are asked to spend no more than five minutes on each question in your viva. This means you will normally cover at least six topics in each one. They will also be aiming to cover all seven areas of competence listed above. Each examiner gives a mark for that viva, and after you have left they average those marks. Following the first viva, a note of areas you have discussed but not the marks is passed on to the second pair of examiners.

When a candidate's marks fall just below an overall pass, the four examiners are asked to reconsider their scores in a 'quartet' at the end of the session and they may be able to alter their mark if they agree that the doctor's performance deserves a pass.

The Practice Experience Questionnaire

The Practice Experience Questionnaire (PEQ), previously known as the log diary, is sent to candidates following application for the exam. It must be completed and returned by a given date so that the examiners will see it before the oral in order to prepare those questions to be based upon it. The questionnaire was extensively revised in 1990, largely to take into account the changes in the GP Contract that year. Although the questionnaire itself is not marked, it is worth preparing in good time and with care.

There are seven sections to be completed:

A. candidate's personal data
B. practice structure
C. practice organisation and facilities
D. workload analysis
E. candidate's own ideas and learning experience
F. clinical diary.

Sections A–D are largely matters of fact and can be filled in with some help from your trainer and practice manager or equivalent.

Sections E and F require a little more thought and preparation. Section E looks at your own ideas and learning. Don't miss this opportunity to introduce areas in which you are keen to answer questions and impress examiners. Section F, the clinical diary, asks for a list of 25 cases seen in the surgery plus 15 home visits and 10 out-of-hours emergencies including 2 night calls where possible. You are asked for the date, patient's initials, age, sex and the main reason for contact. Keep it balanced, but use real patients — they are much easier to remember and you will be uncomfortable on the day if you have done too much 'creative writing'.

Fill in your questionnaire neatly and clearly. Legible handwriting is perfectly acceptable but if you can type it within the rather complex layout, then so much the better. Be sure to keep a copy when you send it off and go through it with a colleague from outside the practice to see which points might be picked up.

It is not unusual for candidates to be sitting the exam when they are between practices or doing short-term locums. In this situation you can either go back to your training practice if you left only recently, or base your questionnaire on another practice in which you have worked lately. If you are working outside general practice then you may need to arrange a locum in order to complete your log.

The first viva

This is based on your PEQ and will therefore focus on practice organisation and discussion of your own patients. You should be able to talk about anything you have mentioned in the questionnaire. You are permitted to take into the exam some notes on the cases you have listed as an aide-memoire. Have your cases numbered as they are on the questionnaire, so that you do not waste time fumbling through pieces of paper. A small notebook with numbered pages or a set of filing cards will create an impression of organisation. It is a good idea to check through the records of your cases shortly before the exam so that you know about subsequent events. The information in the questionnaire is really only to provide the examiners with pegs upon which to hang their questions and the discussion may divert at tangents from time to time. You will not be expected to give clinical round type presentations of your cases but rather to discuss the issues raised by those types of problem you have listed.

The second viva

At the end of 30 minutes in viva 1, a bell rings and discussion stops abruptly. There is a break of approximately 10 minutes during which your first pair of examiners average their marks and pass on a list of topics covered (but not the marks) to the second pair. You will then be directed to your new table. This oral is more free ranging. You will be presented with a mixture of clinical problems and topics from general practice. Questions are often based on experiences of the examiners in their own practice. You may be given a clinical or organisational problem and asked to describe how you might approach it. You may be asked to discuss a lab report, ECG, radiograph, or just about anything you might come across in practice.

Preparation and approach

Try to keep up a steady pace of reading between the written papers and the orals. Because the written papers are set some months before the exam they will inevitably not have covered any very recent 'hot' topics and these may well come up in the viva. Familiarise yourself intimately with your PEQ. The value of practice in viva technique cannot be overstressed. Ask your trainer or any GP who is willing to give you mock oral exams. If you have friends who have taken the exam they can often remember the questions they were asked and try them out on you. If you really want to be scientific then try and video yourself in practice vivas and discuss how you dealt with the questions afterwards.

Many of the skills of viva technique are communication skills. It is of vital importance how you express yourself both verbally and non-verbally. So think about the basics of how you dress, how you speak and how you sit. With practice you can exert a measure of control over the direction in which the questions go. Manoeuvre yourself into areas in which you feel safe to talk and never mention anything you are unable to discuss further.

Revision strategy

There is no 'prescription' for how to prepare yourself for the examination. Each of us has our own approach to study which we vary according to our motivation, strengths and weaknesses, time available and how we feel.

What frightens people about this exam is the sheer breadth of the syllabus. It seems that we need to be experts in all fields of clinical medicine as well as in other areas such as sociology, psychology, epidemiology, law, ethics and business management.

Try not to be daunted. You have actually been preparing for this exam throughout your medical training and your work as a doctor in any context. The breadth of the syllabus should be seen as a bonus. After all, it is the variety within general practice which often attracts us to our chosen career. Also the MRCGP is much less a test of factual knowledge than of attitude and approach, things that we develop throughout our professional and personal development.

You do need to have a good basic knowledge of general practice medicine and some reading will be required. Practise some MCQ papers to identify your areas of weakness and fill in the obvious gaps in your knowledge. For most clinical subjects the books you used as an undergraduate will be sufficiently detailed. The section on further reading at the end of this chapter suggests some sources. The non-clinical facts you need can be found in books but are often better learnt by discussion with trainers and other colleagues and selective reading of a few relevant journals and periodicals.

There does seem to be a particular way of thinking which the examiners are looking for. There is no doubt that you will be at an advantage if you are sitting the examination while you are in the thick of general practice and talking daily with other GPs and trainees. The importance of being part of a half-day release or similar peer group cannot be overestimated. It is almost inevitable that the sort of issues which arise both formally and informally in such a setting are just those which the examiners are likely to be addressing.

REFERENCES

Belton A 1986 How to increase your trainee pass rate in the MRCGP examination. Journal of the Association of Course Organisers 2: 56–64

Lockie C (ed) 1990 Examination for the Royal College of General Practitioners (MRCGP). Occasional Paper 46. RCGP, London

Lowenstein S R, Libby L S, Mountain R D, Hanbrough J F, Hill D M, Scoggin C H 1981 Cardiopulmonary resuscitation by medical and surgical house officers. Lancet 2: 679–681

Pai G R C, Haites N E, Rawles J M 1987 One thousand heart attacks in Grampian; the place of cardiopulmonary resuscitation in general practice. British Medical Journal 294: 352–354

Royal College of General Practitioners 1972 The future general practitioner— learning and teaching. British Medical Journal, London

Sackett D L, Haynes R B, Guyatt G H, Tugwell P 1991 Clinical epidemiology. A basic science for clinical medicine. Little, Brown, Boston

Skinner D V, Camm A J, Myles S 1985 Cardiopulmonary resuscitation skills of preregistration house officers. British Medical Journal 290: 1549–1550

Tombleson P, Wakeford R 1989 Why do trainees take the MRCGP examination? (Correspondence). Journal of the Royal College of General Practitioners 39: 168–171

Vincent R, Martin B, Williams G, Quinn E, Robertson G, Chamberlain D A 1984 A community training scheme in cardiopulmonary resuscitation. British Medical Journal 288: 617–620

Walker J H, Stanley I M, Venables T L, Gambrill E C, Hodgkin G K H 1983 The MRCGP Examination and its methods. 1: Introduction. Journal of the Royal College of General Practitioners 33: 662–665

FURTHER READING — See also Chapter 10

Elliot P 1989 MRCGP MCQs. Springer Verlag, London
Freeling P 1983 A workbook for trainees in general practice. Wright, Bristol
Gambrill E, Moulds A, Fry J, Brooks D 1988 The MRCGP study book. Butterworth/Update, London
Murray T S 1986 Modified essay questions for the MRCGP. Blackwell, Oxford
Palmer K T 1992 Notes for the MRCGP. Blackwell, Oxford
Sandars J E (ed) 1985 MRCGP practice exams. Pastest, Hemel Hempstead

Appendix I (Reproduced with permission from Walker et al 1983)

A. 1. Clinical practice —health and disease

The candidate will be required to demonstrate a knowledge of the diagnosis, management and, where appropriate, the prevention of diseases of importance in general practice.
a. The range of the normal
b. The patterns of illness
c. The natural history of diseases
d. Prevention
e. Early diagnosis
f. Diagnostic methods and techniques
g. Management and treatment

2. Clinical practice — human development

The candidate will be expected to possess a knowledge of human development and be able to demonstrate the value of this knowledge in the diagnosis and management of patients in general practice.
a. Genetics
b. Fetal development
c. Physical development in childhood, maturity and ageing
d. Intellectual development in childhood, maturity and ageing
e. Emotional development in childhood, maturity and ageing
f. The range of the normal

3. Clinical practice — human behaviour

The candidate must demonstrate an understanding of human behaviour particularly as it affects the presentation and management of disease.
a. Behaviour presenting to a general practitioner
b. Behaviour in interpersonal relationships
c. Behaviour of the family
d. Behaviour in the doctor-patient relationship

4. Medicine and society

The candidate must be familiar with the common sociological and epidemiological concepts and their relevance to medical care and demonstrate a knowledge of the organisation of medical and related services in the United Kingdom and abroad.
a. Sociological aspects of health and illness
b. The uses of epidemiology
c. The organisation of medical care in the United Kingdom — comparisons with other countries
d. The relationship of medical services to other institutions of society
e. Ethics
f. Historical perspectives of general practice

5. The practice

The candidate must demonstrate a knowledge of practice organisation and administration and be able critically to discuss recent developments in the evolution of general practice.
a. Practice management
b. The team
c. Financial matters
d. Premises and equipment
e. Medical records
f. Medicolegal matters
g. Research

B. The examination is designed to assess in a variety of ways the skills of the candidate in:

a. Interpersonal communication
b. History taking and information gathering
c. Selecting examinations using investigations and procedures
d. Recording information
e. Interpreting information
f. Problem definition and hypothesis formation
g. Early diagnosis
h. Defining the range of intervention
i. Selecting therapy
j. Providing continuing care
k. Interventive and preventive medicine in relation to: the patient, the family, and the community
l. The organisation of his practice and himself
m. Teamwork, delegation, and in relating to other colleagues
n. Business methods
o. Communications

C. The candidate will be expected to demonstrate appropriate attitudes to his patients, his colleagues and to the role of the general practitioner. He must demonstrate his ability to develop and extend his knowledge and skills through continuing education.

Appendix II

CRITICAL READING CRIB

Phase 1— Quick overview

Source	Is the article from a well-known, peer-reviewed journal?
Title	What does the title say?
	Does it relate to content?
	Is it interesting?
	Does it have credibility?
Authors	How many?
	Where are they working?
	Are they known?
	What is their background?
Acknowledgements	May be of interest to see who supported the study.
References	May locate the paper in a 'tradition'.
	What period do they cover?
Abstract	This is not provided in the CRQ paper. Under normal circumstances, however, it would give you an overall idea of the paper and help you decide whether to read on. Does it accurately describe the paper?

Phase 2 — Reading the paper in detail

Introduction	Is the scene clearly set?
	What is the 'question'?
	Is the literature review comprehensive and does it relate to the 'question'?
	Are the aims and objectives of the study clear?
Method	What kind of study is it?
	• Descriptive (cross-sectional).
	• Retrospective (case-control).
	• Prospective (longitudinal/cohort).
	• Trial (intervention/experimental study).
	• Natural experiment.
	Was there a pilot study?
	Is the *sample*:
	• appropriate size?
	• randomised?
	• unbiased?
	• divided into comparison groups?
	Is sufficient detail of method given for others to replicate the study?
	How were the results *analysed?*
Results	Should present results only.
	What was the response rate?
	Are tables clear and accurate?
	Are statistical tests appropriate?
Discussion	An overview should be given of method and results:
	• critique of method
	• discussion of results
	• interpretation of findings.
	A conclusion should state whether the question is answered and comment on the generalisability of the result, placing it in the context of the literature review. The next step should be suggested, i.e. where do we go from here?

9. Diplomas for trainees

Joe Rosenthal

INTRODUCTION

As we have said in the previous chapter, there are pros and cons to pursuing further qualifications as a trainee. The following are the most popular diplomas taken. None of them is compulsory for gaining an eventual partnership in general practice. Entrance fees are not given below as these will change from year to year. Regulations for entry and examination formats may also change from the time of writing and so should be checked with the appropriate examining board when you are thinking of applying.

There is a lot to be said for entering a diploma examination shortly after you have completed a post in the specialty concerned so that the approach is fresh in your mind. In order to prepare for clinical parts of exams there is no better way than to see patients and discuss them afterwards with a friendly registrar or consultant. Several centres run courses to help prepare candidates for each of these examinations. Ask locally for those available and keep an eye on the advertisements in the BMJ. Courses which offer practice in both written and clinical components of the exams are strongly recommended.

The Diploma of the Royal College of Obstetricians and Gynaecologists (DRCOG)

This is probably the most popular diploma taken by GP trainees. This is because most trainees do complete a 6-month post in obstetrics and gynaecology and there is also a feeling that, since eligibility for the FHSA obstetric list tends to be a desirable attribute when applying for partnerships, it may improve potential job prospects. In fact, the criteria for admission to the obstetric list (i.e. those GPs who are eligible for a higher rate of payment for the provision of maternity services) in the Red Book do not include possession of the diploma, but rather the completion of a 6-month post in an appropriate unit (among other possibilities).

The diploma is intended to recognise a general practitioner's interest in obstetrics and gynaecology and is not a specialist qualification.

The Royal College of Obstetricians and Gynaecologists produces a booklet entitled *Diploma Examination Regulations* which can be obtained from the following address:

The Examination Secretary
Royal College of Obstetricians and Gynaecologists
27 Sussex Place
Regents Park
LONDON NW1 4RG
Telephone: 071-262 5425

The examination is at present held twice a year, in April/May and October/November. Check closing dates for entry with the College. There is a choice between London and selected provincial centres for the written paper, but the locations of clinicals and vivas are decided by the College.

The number of attempts at this examination is limited to five.

Eligibility

The regulations state that:

1. The candidate must be fully registered as a medical practitioner in the register maintained by the General Medical Council or the Medical Council of Ireland.

2. Application must be made on the appropriate form by the given closing date.

3. The candidate must have held a recognised appointment for 6 consecutive months and completed that appointment by the closing date for receipt of entries. (Recognised appointments are limited to the United Kingdom, Republic of Ireland, and HM Forces. Part-time training may be permitted with advance approval of the College.)

To confirm eligibility, return the form you receive from the College with the examination regulations, together with two certificates confirming your recognised appointment, and your medical registration. Possession of the Joint Committee on Contraception Certificate in General Family Planning is no longer a requirement for entry to the Diploma. (A new diploma in Family Planning is being developed by the Royal College of Obstetricians and Gynaecologists.)

Examination format

The examination itself comprises three parts:

1. *Written paper*. This has two sections:
    a. a multiple-choice question paper lasting 75 minutes
    b. an essay paper lasting 90 minutes during which two compulsory questions are to be answered.

2. *Clinical examination.* 20 minutes with a patient followed by discussion of the case with examiners. You may be presented with an obstetric, gynaecological or family planning patient.

3. *Oral examination.* 20 minute viva which may cover any aspect of obstetrics, gynaecology or related subjects.

Syllabus

The detailed syllabus is available from the College and includes a broad range of topics in obstetrics, gynaecology, neonatal medicine and family planning.

Recommended reading the DRCOG

Rymer J, Davis G, Rodin A, Chapman C 1990 Preparation and revision for the DRCOG. Churchill Livingstone, Edinburgh

Stirrat G M 1987 Aids to obstetrics and gynaecology for MRCOG, Part 2. Churchill Livingstone, Edinburgh

---

Copies of past examination papers are available from the College.

The Diploma in Child Health (DCH)

This examination is administered by the Royal College of Physicians of London. It is generally regarded as a more difficult examination than the DRCOG. It is held twice a year. The majority of entrants will have had 6 months' experience in a paediatrics post, either in hospital or the community, but you can enter on the basis of experience working with children in general practice itself.

The DCH is designed to give recognition of competence in the care of children and not to test detailed knowledge of the inpatient care, nor minutiae of management of rare conditions. The aim is to test primary care paediatrics. The number of attempts is limited to four.

The Regulations for the DCH are available from the Royal College of Physicians at the following address:

The Examination Department
Royal College of Physicians
11 St Andrew's Place
Regents Park
LONDON NW1 4LE
Telephone: 071 935 1174

Eligibility

1. Candidates must hold a recognised medical qualification.

2. 12 months' experience in the care of children is recommended but not obligatory.

Examination format

The examination itself comprises two sections:

1. Written section. This has two parts:
    - paper 1 — three hours to complete 10 short note questions and two case commentaries.
    - paper 2 — two hours to complete 60 multiple choice questions.
2. Clinical section. Consisting of:
    - one long case — 40 minutes with a patient followed by 25 minutes with the examiners.
    - several short cases — 25 minutes, of which 10 minutes will be devoted to developmental testing.

Candidates must pass the multiple choice question paper in order to attend the clinical section.

Syllabus

The detailed syllabus is available from the Royal College of Physicians and includes all aspects of paediatrics relevant to the primary care setting.

Recommended reading for the DCH

Harvey D, Kovar I 1991 Child health: a textbook for the DCH. Churchill Livingstone, Edinburgh
Hull D, Johnston D 1981 Essential paediatrics. Churchill Livingstone, Edinburgh
Hull D, Polnay L 1988 Community paediatrics. Churchill Livingstone, Edinburgh
Modell M, Boyd R 1988 Paediatric problems in general practice. Oxford University Press, Oxford

---

Copies of past examination papers are available from the Royal College of Physicians.

The Diploma in Community Child Health (DCCH)

This examination is administered by the Royal College of Physicians of Edinburgh, the Royal College of General Practitioners and the Faculty of Public Health Medicine of the Royal Colleges of Physicians of the United Kingdom (referred to as the participating bodies). There is inevitably considerable overlap with the DCH but the emphasis is much more on the community aspects of child health, and so will probably appeal to doctors with experience either as an SHO in community paediatrics or as a clinical medical officer.

The regulations for the DCCH are available from the Royal College of Physicians of Edinburgh at the following address:

The Registrar, Royal College of Physicians, 9 Queen Street, EDINBURGH EH2 1JQ (Telephone: 031 225 7324).

Eligibility

The regulations state that:

1. Candidates must hold qualifications in medicine, surgery, and obstetrics and gynaecology that are approved by the participating bodies. Detailed evidence is required that at the time of examination they will have held a medical qualification for at least two years.

2. A testimonial is required, signed by a Member or Fellow of a Royal College or Faculty to certify that the candidate will, at the time of the examination, have acquired the knowledge, skills and attitudes outlined in the 'core curriculum' for the examination.

Examination format

1. A modified essay question lasting one and a quarter hours and containing 6–10 sequential questions, all of which must be answered.
2. 10–20 short answer questions to be completed in one and a half hours.
3. Written examination lasting 45 minutes on projected material which may be still transparencies or moving cine film or videotape.
4. An objective structured clinical examination lasting 45–60 minutes and comprising short tests of the candidate's ability to solve problems, interpret information, communicate, examine and manage a patient and his or her parents.

Syllabus

The detailed 'core curriculum' is available from the Royal College of Physicians of Edinburgh, and covers all aspects of community child health. Past papers and a detailed reading list can also be obtained from the College.

Recommended reading for the DCCH

As for DCH recommendations plus:
Department of Health 1992 Immunisation against infectious disease. HMSO, London
Hall D M B 1989 Health for all children: a programme for child health surveillance. Oxford University Press, Oxford
Illingworth R S 1983 Development of the infant and young child. Churchill Livingstone, Edinburgh

The Diploma in Geriatric Medicine (DGM)

This examination is conducted by the Royal College of Physicians and is held twice a year. It is designed to give recognition of competence in the provision of care for the elderly to GPs, vocational trainees, clinical assistants and other doctors with interests in or responsibilities for the care of elderly people but not working in consultant career posts in departments of geriatric medicine. The number of attempts is limited to four.

The regulations for the DGM are available from the Royal College of Physicians in London (address given in section on DCH above).

Eligibility

The regulations state that:

1. Candidates must hold a recognised medical qualification.
2. Eligible candidates must:

   either (i) have held a post approved for professional training in a department specialising in the care of the elderly, and provide certification from the consultant in charge of the department where the post was held

   or (ii) have had experience over a period of two years since full registration in which the care of the elderly formed a significant part

   or (iii) have been appointed as a principal in general practice before January 1990.

Examination format

1. *Written section*:

   - paper 1 (3 hours) — short-note questions. There are five sections, each containing five items from which four must be answered. A 'short note' answer should be of the order of 100 words.
   - paper 2 (3 hours) — essay questions. The paper contains two sections. The first comprises four questions concerned with systematic knowledge of which one compulsory and one other question should be attempted. Section 2 contains four questions concerned with management of clinical problems of which one compulsory question and two others should be attempted.

2. *Clinical section*. This comprises:

   - one long case — 45 minutes for interviewing and examining the patient, and 30 minutes with the examiners.
   - short-case examination — 20 minutes. Candidates will be assessed on several items which may include short cases, audiovisual material, results of investigations, equipment and appliances.

Syllabus

The detailed syllabus is available from the Royal College of Physicians of London. The emphasis is placed on ability to synthesise understanding of the manifestation and course of age-associated impairments common in old age with knowledge of the health and social services available in order to identify appropriate plans of management and referral.

> Recommended reading for the DGM
>
> Bennett G C, Ebrahim S 1992 The essentials of health care of the elderly. Edward Arnold, London
> Thompson M K 1990 Commonsense geriatrics. Clinical Press, Bristol
> Wilcock G K, Gray J A M, Longmore J M 1991 Geriatric problems in general practice. Oxford University Press, Oxford
>
> The journal Geriatric Medicine is particularly useful. Refer especially to a series of articles entitled 'Diploma coach' which were run in 1989.

Copies of past examination papers are available from the Royal College of Physicians.

CONCLUSION

As we have said, the diplomas detailed above are those which are most popular amongst trainees. Many other qualifications are available, depending on your experience and plans. Trainees planning to work in developing countries, for example, may consider the Diploma in Tropical Medicine and Hygiene (DTM&H), or those with the appropriate experience may sit the Diploma in Anaesthetics. Whatever your interest, it is likely that there is some qualification which you can acquire. Our advice is that these should be considered if they will provide a means to an end, rather than as an end in themselves.

10. Further reading

Joe Rosenthal

The trainee year is the end of the beginning of general practice education. Where do we go from here? The breadth and rate of change in the discipline make it essential that we continue to learn throughout our working lives. But learning is not simply the acquisition of knowledge, and continuing education is not just 'keeping up-to-date'. We need to carry on learning in order to remain stimulated and enjoy our work. In this way we benefit not just ourselves but our patients and the people with whom we work.

Numerous and varied learning opportunities are available to us in such forms as magazines, journals, audiotapes, videotapes, seminars, practitioners' groups, lectures and courses. But the most valuable sources of education are our colleagues and our patients in day-to-day practice.

The list of books that follows is presented as a 'menu' to sample according to your taste and appetite. All the texts are general and widely considered to be of value in their particular areas. Some may be worth reading in their entirety, others for selective use depending on your needs. The categories are, to some extent, arbitrary and will often overlap. We have not included clinical references although some of the works listed as general reading cover clinical matters.

Apart from some early titles which are thought of as classic and still of relevance, the majority of suggestions are recent and all are readily available at the time of writing.

GENERAL READING

Berger J, Mohr P 1967 A fortunate man. Penguin, London
Berne E 1970 Games people play. Penguin, London
Cronin A J 1939 The citadel. Gollancz
Helman C G 1984 Culture, health and illness. Wright, London
Hodgkin K 1985 Towards earlier diagnosis: a guide to primary care. Churchill Livingstone, Edinburgh
Huygen F J A 1978 Family medicine: the medical life history of families. Dekker & Vandervegt, Nijmegen, Netherlands (Republished 1990 RCGP)
McPherson A 1990 Women's problems in general practice. Oxford University Press, Oxford
McWhinney I R 1989 A textbook of family medicine. Oxford University Press, Oxford
Munthe A 1929 The story of San Michele. John Murray,
Orwell G 1949 Down and out in London and Paris. Secker & Warburg
Shaw G B 1946 Mrs Warren's profession. In: Plays unpleasant. Penguin, London

Stott P 1983 Milestones. Pan, London (Republished 1991 RCGP)
Widgery D 1992 Some lives! A GP's East End. Sinclair Stevenson, London

THE CONSULTATION

Balint M 1957 The doctor, his patient and the illness. Churchill Livingstone, Edinburgh
Byrne P, Long B 1976 Doctors talking to patients. HMSO, London
Neighbour R 1987 The inner consultation. MTP, Lancaster
Pendleton D, Schofield T, Tate P, Havelock P 1989 The consultation. An approach to learning and teaching Oxford University Press, Oxford
Tuckett D, Boulton M, Olsen C, Williams A 1985 Meetings between experts: an approach to sharing ideas in medical consultations. Tavistock, London

EPIDEMIOLOGY AND STATISTICS

Bland M 1987 An introduction to medical statistics. Oxford University Press, Oxford
Morrell D 1988 Epidemiology in general practice. Oxford University Press, Oxford
Pickles W 1939 Epidemiology in a country practice. Wright, Bristol (Republished 1984 RCGP)
Sackett D, Hayes R B, Guyatt G H, Tugwell P 1991 Clinical epidemiology: a basic science for clinical medicine. Little, Brown, Boston

MEDICAL ETHICS

British Medical Association 1988 Philosophy and practice of medical ethics. BMA, London
Campbell A V 1984 Moderated care, A theology of professional care. SPCK
Campbell A V, Higgs R 1982 In that case. Medical ethics in everyday practice. Darton, Longman & Todd, London
Gillon R 1985 Philosophical medical ethics. Wiley, Chichester

MRCGP EXAMINATION

Elliot P 1989 MRCGP MCQs. Springer Verlag, London
Freeling P 1983 A workbook for trainees in general practice. Wright, Bristol
Gambrill E, Moulds A, Fry J, Brooks D 1988 The MRCGP study book. Butterworth Update, London
Murray T S 1986 Modified essay questions for the MRCGP. Blackwell, Oxford
Palmer K T 1992 Notes for the MRCGP. Blackwell, Oxford
Sandars J E (ed) 1985 MRCGP practice exams. Pastest, Hemel Hempstead

PRACTICE MANAGEMENT

Bolden K, Lewis A, Sawyer B 1992 Practice management. Blackwell, Oxford
Chisholm J (ed) 1990 Making sense of the new contract. Radcliffe, Oxford
Hasler J, Bryceland C, Hobden-Clarke L, Rose P 1991 Handbook of practice management. Churchill Livingstone, Edinburgh

PREVENTION

Lock S (ed) 1983 Practising prevention. BMA, London
Priest V, Speller V 1991 Risk factor management manual. Radcliffe, Oxford

RESEARCH AND AUDIT

Armstrong D, Calnan M, Grace J 1990 Research methods for general practitioners. Oxford University Press, Oxford
Howie J G R 1989 Research in general practice. Chapman Hill, London
Irvine D, Irvine S (eds) 1991 Making sense of audit. Radcliffe, Oxford
Marinker M (ed) 1991 Medical audit in general practice. BMA, London

SOCIAL SCIENCES

Armstrong D 1989 An outline of sociology as applied to medicine. Wright, London
Patrick D, Scambler G (eds) 1986 Sociology as applied to medicine. Balliere Tindall, Guildford
Shillitoe R W 1988 Psychology and diabetes. Chapman & Hall, London
Weinmann J 1987 An outline of psychology as applied to medicine. Wright, London

Index

Accidents
　major, 21
　prevention, 184–7
Accountability, 63
Active listening, 118–20
Activities of daily living, 225
Advertising
　by drug industry, 88
　practice leaflet, 63
Advice
　giving effective, 122–4
　within consultation, 55–7
Agendas, 111–12
Alcohol, 168–70
　population strategies, 146
　and psychiatric problems, 229
Allowances, social security, 211, 212, 217
Angry patients, 126–7
Annual reports, 64
Antibiotics, 195–7
Antonovsky, A., 33, 34
Anxiety, 226–8
　and dyspepsia, 199
Appointments system, 52
Asher, R., 35
Assertiveness, 129–33
Assessment, 16–17
Associate Advisor, 4, 17
Asthma
　care in practice, 184
　clinics, 56
Audit, 255–63

Back pain, 201–3
Bad news, breaking, 125–6, 219
Balance sheet, 90, 103–4
Balint, Michael, 114
Barron, F., 39
Behaviour
　illness behaviour, 191–2
　modification, 218–19
Beliefs, 191–2
　Rosenstock's health belief model, 154–5
Benefits, social security, 211, 212, 217

Bereavement, 41
　emotional adjustment to handicapped child, 218
Breast cancer, 177–80
British Association of Immediate Care Schemes (BASICS), 21
British Diabetic Association, 232
British Heart Foundation, 174
British Regional Heart Study, 171–2
　GP score (Shaper score), 175–6
Budgets, practice, 83–6

CAGE questionnaire, 169
Capitation fees, 91
Car allowance, 6
Carers, 211–12
　prevention of mental ill-health, 229
　see also Community care
Cartwright, A., 37–8
Case mix, 11
Certificate in cardiopulmonary resuscitation (CPR), 269
Certificate in child health surveillance (CHS), 269
Certificate of satisfactory completion, 16, 19
Certification forms, 100
Cervical screening, 151–3
　target payments, 92
Chieseman, W. E., 39
Child health surveillance, 59, 162–4
　certificate, 269
　evaluation, 163
　fees, 162
Children
　health promotion, 161–5
　mental handicap, 217
Cholesterol, 145–6, 171–2
Chronic disease, 209–34
　coping strategies, 210
　home visits, 213
　management clinics, 56
　monitoring (tertiary prevention), 139, 183–4
Claim forms, 100–101

295

INDEX

Clinical care, 189–235
  continuing, 209–34
  episodic, 190–208
Clinical decision making, 192–4
Clinical epidemiology, 194
Clinical protocols, 213
Communication skills, 11–12, 105–35
  doctors, 106–10
  health education, 156–7
  information and advice, 122–4
  listening, 118–20
  monitoring, 107
  non-verbal cues, 121–2
  role play, 108
  style, 116–17
  touch, 122
Community care
  mental handicap, 214–20
  psychiatric problems, 228
  see also Carers
Community Care Act (1993), 214
Community Mental Handicap Team, 217
Computers, 62, 77–9
  Data Protection Act, 62, 78
  literature searches, 242
Confidentiality, 75
  computers, 62, 78
  research, 252
Congenital rubella syndrome, 165
Consultations, 39–42
  appointments system, 52
  communication skills, 106–25
  communication style, 116–17
  doctor's tasks, 109
  GP Contract requirements, 51–5
  health advice, 55–7
  health education, 156–7
  length, 115
  patients, 110–12
  routine surgeries, 10–11
  setting, 50, 112–14
  starting surgeries, 9–10
  telephone, 53
  theory, 114–18
Continuing care, 209–34
Contraceptive services, 58–9
  fees, 92
  forms, 100
Contracts
  of employment, trainees, 5–7
  GP Contract see GP Contract (1990)
  purchasing, 82–3
Coping strategies
  chronic illness, 210
  trainees, 21
Coronary heart disease
  prevention, 56–7, 170–77
  protective factors, 171
  risk factors, 145–7, 170–73, 175–6
Coronary Prevention Group, 174

Action Plan, 175
Counselling, 228, 229
Course organiser, 17
Crisis intervention, 229
Cultural influences, 110

Data collection, 246–51
Data Protection Act, 62, 78
Day care, 220
Decision making, 192–4
Delegation
  deputising services, 54–5
  practice nurses see Practice nurses
  practice staff, 75
  recalls, 61
Depression, 226–8
Deprivation payments, 94
Deputising services, 54–5
Diabetes, 230–34
  clinics, 56
  GP's learning needs, 233
  patient education, 231–2
Diploma in Child Health (DCH), 285–6
Diploma in Community Child Health (DCCH), 286–7
Diploma in Geriatric Medicine (DGM), 287–9
Diploma of the Royal College of Obstetricians and Gynaecologists (DRCOG), 283–5
Diplomas, 283–9
Disability, 209–10
  economic disadvantage, 211
Disease prevention see Prevention of disease
Dispensing, 62–3
District Health Authorities, 81–3
Doctors' and Dentists' Review Body, 89
Down's syndrome, 215–16
Drugs
  clinical trials, 244–5
  older people, 222–4
  prescribing see Prescribing
Dundee Risk Score, 175
Dyspepsia, 198–201

Education, GP
  GP Contract requirements, 64–6
  and prescribing of drugs, 88
Education, health see Health education
Elderly patients see Older patients
Emergencies, 204–8
  experience of, 12
  handling on-call, 11
  psychiatric, 205–8
Employment
  GP Contract see GP Contract (1990)
  part-time outside practice hours, 6
  trainees contract, 5–7

INDEX

Endoscopy, 200
Environment, 36–7
Epidemiology, clinical, 194
Epilepsy, 210
Episodic illness, 190–208
Equipment, 21–2, 76–9
Ethics
  health education, 158
  health promotion, 157–8
  research, 252
  screening, 157
Eye contact, 122

Facilitators, 161
Family Health Services Authority (FHSA), 79–83
  Medical Audit Advisory Groups, 257
  organisation, 80
  patients' records, 61–2
  role, 79–83
  Statement of Fees and Allowances, 6, 89
  visits to, 8
Fees
  capitation, 91
  child health surveillance, 162
  claim forms, 100–101
  contraceptive services, 92
  deprivation payments, 94
  health promotion clinics, 56, 92
  items of service, 91–2
  list of fees and allowances, 102
  miscellaneous forms, 93
  out-of-hours work, 54–5, 91
  Statement of Fees and Allowances (Red Book), 6, 89
  vaccinations, 57
  see also Pay
Financing
  practices, 81–6
  provision of care, 79–94
  research, 253–4
Fitness, physical, 32
Forms, 100–101
Framingham Heart Study, 171
Freud, Sigmund, 42
Functional capacity, 32–3
Funding *see* Financing

General health checks, 153
General Medical Council (GMC) Trainee Committee, 19
General practice *see* Practices
Government policy
  Health of the Nation, 56–7, 142–3, 166
  prevention of disease, 143–4
  smoking, 166–7
GP Contract (1990), 9, 50–66
  additional services, 58–60

GP education, 64–6
  main requirements, 51
  over-75s, 60, 224–5
  personal medical services, 51–8
  prevention of disease, 144
  recalls, 60–61
  records and reports, 61–4

Half-day release scheme, 19–20
Handicap, 209–10
  mental, 214–20
Hardiness, 33–5
Health
  as absence of disease or illness, 28–30
  as adaptation to environment, 36–7
  attitudes to, 38–9
  concepts/descriptions of, 28–37
  and happiness, 45
  healthy life style, 166–70
  as normality, 30–31
  relation to illness, 37–9
  resources for, 40
  and socioeconomic factors, 143
  of trainee, 20–21
  as wellbeing, 31–5
  World Health Organization definition, 28, 35–6, 138
Health advice
  giving effective, 122–4
  within consultation, 55–7
Health care evaluation (audit), 255–63
Health checks, general, 153
Health education, 154–7
  definition, 139
  ethics, 158
  prevention of accidents, 186
Health of the Nation, 56–7, 142–3, 166
Health promotion
  childhood, 161–5
  clinics, 12, 56, 92
  definition, 137–8
  ethics, 157–8
  GP as resource for, 42–4
  high-risk strategy, 145–7
  model, 139
  opportunities in general practice, 145
  population strategy, 145–7
  practice organisation, 159–61
  role of primary health care team, 144–5, 159
Health protection, 139–40
Heart-sink patients, 41
Home visits, 53–4
  to chronically ill, 213
  requests for, 127–8, 204
Howie, John, 193, 194, 196
Hypertension, 180–83

Illness behaviour, 191–2

Immunisation *see* Vaccination
Impairment, 209
Independent living, 221
Index Medicus, 241–2
Indicative Prescribing Amount, 87
Indicative Prescribing Scheme, 86–7, 89
Indigestion, 198–201
Information, giving effective, 122–4
Insurance
  equipment, 22
  practice nurses, 58
  trainees, 7, 21
Interview expenses, 7
Intuition, 109
Items of service, 91–2

Jargon, 123
Joint Committee for Postgraduate Training in General Practice (JCPTGP), 17–18
Journals
  critical reading, 275, 282
  publication in, 254–5
  research resources, 241–3

Kobasa, S. C., 34

Leaflets
  explanatory, 123, 126
  health education, 157
  practice, 63
Learning
  methods, 22
  objectives, 5
Letters to hospital consultants *see* Referrals
Libraries, 241–2
Life style
  and dyspepsia, 199
  healthy, 166–70
  modification, 172–3
Listening skills, 118–20
Literature searches, 241–2
Local knowledge, 9

Mackenzie, Sir James, 237
Major accident equipment, 21
Mammography, 178–80
Management skills, 14–15, 133–4
Marital problems, 229
Maternity leave, 7
Maternity medical services, 58–9
Measles, mumps, rubella (MMR) vaccine, 165
Medical Audit Advisory Groups, 257
Medical bags, 21–2
Medication *see* Drugs; Prescribing

Medico-legal problems, 18–19
  records, 61–2
MEDLINE, 242
Mental handicap, 214–20
Mental Health Act (1983), 205–8
Mental illness, 226–30
Minor surgery services, 59
Monitoring
  communication skills, 107
  disease (tertiary prevention), 139, 183–4
  provision of care, 79–94
Morbidity, 141–2
Mortality, 141–2, 143
MRCGP examination, 267–81
  application, 268–9
  critical reading question paper (CRQ), 274–6, 282
  eligibility, 268
  format, 270
  modified essay question paper (MEQ), 272–4
  multiple choice question paper (MCQ), 270–72
  oral examination, 276–7
  Practice Experience Questionnaire, 276, 277–8
  revision strategy, 279–80
  syllabus, 268, 281
  vivas, 278–9
Multiphasic screening, 153
Multiple Risk Factor Intervention Trial (MRFIT), 172

National Health Service Breast Screening Programme, 179
Negotiating skills, 132–3
Neighbour, Roger, 116
Non-verbal communication, 121–2
Normality, 30–31
North of England Study of Standards and Performance in General Practice (1992), 262
North Karalia Study, 172

Older patients, 220–26
  over-75s, 60, 224–5
Out-of-hours work (on-call duties), 11, 54–5
  fees, 54–5, 91

Paperwork, 9
Partnerships, 22–3
Pathology services, 84
Patients
  angry, 126–7
  beliefs and behaviour, 191–2
  consultations, 110–12

Patients (*contd*)
  frequent attenders, 41
  newly registered, 60
  older, 220–26
  over-75s, 60, 224–5
  records *see* Records
  telephone calls *see* Telephones
Pay
  General Practitioners, 89–90, 93–4
  Postgraduate Education Allowance, 64–6
  practice nurses, 58
  sick pay, 7
  staff, 70–71, 90
  of trainees, 6–7
  see also Fees
Peckham Health Centre, 27, 29, 140
Physical fitness, 32
Pickles, William, 237
Postgraduate Education Allowance (PGEA), 64–6
Practice Experience Questionnaire, 276, 277–8
Practice leaflet, 63
Practice managers, 72–3
Practice nurses
  health education, 156
  health promotion, 56
  insurance, 58
  pay, 58
  prevention of disease, 161
  recalls, 61
  role within the team, 133
  vaccinations, 57–8
Practices
  approval for training, 95–6
  budgets, 83–6
  choosing, 3–5
  expenses, 90
  fundholding, 81–3, 83–6
  location, 4, 66–7
  organisation, 159–61
  receipts, 91–3
  relationships within the team, 133–4
  trainers *see* Trainers
Prejudice, 121
Premises, 66–9
Prescribing, 62–3, 86–9
  accountability, 63
  antibiotics, 195–7
  dyspepsia, 201
  funding, 85
  Indicative Prescribing Amount, 87
  Indicative Prescribing Scheme, 86–7, 89
  patterns, 88–9
  Prescribing Analysis and Cost (PACT), 87–8
  Prescription Pricing Authority (PPA), 87
Prevention of accidents, 184–7
Prevention of disease, 40
  breast cancer, 178
  coronary heart disease, 56–7, 170–77
  definition, 137–8
  ethics, 157–8
  facilitators, 161
  Government policies, 143–4, 166–7
  GP Contract, 144
  handicap, 217–18
  high-risk strategy, 145–7
  hypertension, 181–2
  mental illness, 229
  older people, 224–5
  opportunities in general practice, 145
  population strategy, 145–7, 167
  practice organisation, 159–61
  preventive care cards, 159–60
  primary, 138
  role of primary health care team, 144–5, 159
  scope for, 141–2
  secondary *see* Screening
  socioeconomic factors, 143
  strategies, 141–7
  tertiary (monitoring), 139, 183–4
Primary health care team, 73–5
  and alcohol, 168–9
  role in prevention of accidents, 186–7
  role in prevention of disease/health promotion, 144–5, 159
  and smoking, 167
Private income, 93
Protocols
  clinical, 213
  research, 252–3
Psychiatry, 226–30
  emergencies, 205–8
  referrals, 228–9
Purchasing of health services, 81–3, 83–6

Quality of care, 255–63
Questionnaires, 247–9

Recalls, 60–61
Receptionists, 8, 69
  job description, 99
  role within the team, 133
  training, 71–2
Records
  FHSA, 61–2
  forms, 100
  GP Contract requirements, 61–4
  medico-legal problems, 61–2
  parent-held, 163
  patient-held, 123–4, 161
  prevention of disease/health promotion, 159–61
  of telephone conversations, 129
  vaccinations, 58
Red Book, 6, 89

Referrals
    appropriateness, 193
    letters, 134
    psychiatric problems, 228–9
Regional Advisor, 4, 17–18
Regional Education Board, 19
Regional GP Postgraduate Committee, 17, 19
Regional Postgraduate Dean, 19
Regional Trainees Committee, 19
Registration forms, 100
Removal expenses, 6
Research, 237–55
    ethics, 252
    funding, 253–4
    literature searches, 241–2
    protocols, 252–3
    publication, 254–5
    study design, 243–51
Residential care, 219–20
Resilience, 33–5
Resistance, 33–5
Responsibilities of trainee, 20–22
Risk factors
    breast cancer, 178
    coronary heart disease, 145–7, 170–73, 175–6
Road traffic accidents, 185
Rosenstock's health belief model, 154–5
Royal College of General Practitioners
    Care of Old People, 221
    diabetes information pack, 230
    Information Resource Centre, 242
    MRCGP examination *see* MRCGP examination
    prevention of disease/health promotion, 144
    Quality Initiatives, 257
    Second National Study (1971–2), 226
Ryle, J. A., 30

Safety
    on-call, 54–5
    psychiatric emergencies, 205
Salaries *see* Pay
Sampling, 245–6
Screening (secondary prevention), 138, 147–54, 177–83
    breast cancer, 177–80
    cervical, 151–3
    ethics, 157
    hypertension, 180–83
    multiphasic, 153
    over-75s, 60, 224–5
Self-awareness, developing, 108
Self-esteem, 44
Seven Countries Study, 171
Shaper score, 175–6
Sick pay, 7
Smoking, 166–8

coronary heart disease, 171–2, 175–6
and ulcers, 199
Social security benefits, 211, 212, 217
Social support, 43–4
Social workers, 205–6
Socioeconomic factors
    and dyspepsia, 199
    and health, 143
Sore throat, 195–8
Staff, 69–76
    delegation to, 75
    full-time, 71
    morale, 76
    practice managers, 72–3
    practice nurses *see* Practice nurses
    prevention of disease, 161
    receptionists *see* Receptionists
    salaries, 70–71, 90
    training, 71
Standardised mortality ratio (SMR), 143
Statement of Fees and Allowances (Red Book), 6, 89
Stigma, 209–10
Stress
    and dyspepsia, 199
    trainees, 21
Stroke, 180–81
Study design, 243–51
Study leave, 20
Surgeries *see* Consultations
Symptoms, 190–91

Targets
    Health of the Nation, 142
    payments, 92
    prevention of accidents, 184
    vaccinations, 57–8, 92, 165
Teamwork, 133–4
Telephones
    consultations, 53
    conversations with patients, 127–9
    requests for emergency visits, 127–8, 204
Terminal illness, 40
Theses, 255
Touch, 122
Tracer conditions, 232–3
Trainee year, 3–23
Trainers
    approval for training, 95–6
    communicating with, 129–33
    initial contact, 4–5
    problems with, 17–18
    shadowing, 8, 9
    as source of help, 17
    trainer/trainee relationship, 4, 14
    training course, 96
    view of training and practice, 5
Training requirements, 95–6
Tutorials, 5

Ulcers, peptic, 198–201

Vaccination, 57–8, 164–5
  fees, 57
  measles, mumps, rubella, 165
  records, 58
  targets, 57–8, 92, 165
  uptake rates, 164–5
Visit requests, 127–8, 204
Vocational training scheme, 7

Walton, Izaak, 45
Wellbeing, 31–5
Whooping cough, 164
Women trainees, 11
Workload
  appointments system, 52
  of trainee, 5
World Health Organization
  definition of health, 28, 35–6, 138
  immunisation aims, 164